Nourishing Dietary Guide for Renal Reset.

Cookbook with Kidney-Friendly Recipes for Optimal Health and Well-being.

By

Candice Foster

TABLE OF CONTENTS

INTRODUCTION

In the realm of health and wellness, few aspects are as crucial as understanding and nurturing the intricate balance of our internal systems. Among these, the health of our kidneys stands paramount, serving as the unsung heroes filtering and purifying our blood, maintaining fluid balance, and regulating electrolytes. As we embark on a journey toward optimal well-being, the significance of a nourishing dietary guide for renal reset becomes not just apparent but imperative.

Enter the "Nourishing Dietary Guide for Renal Reset: Cookbook with Kidney-Friendly Recipes for Optimal Health and Well-being," a comprehensive treasure trove of culinary wisdom designed to harmonize with the unique needs of our renal function. This guide transcends the conventional cookbook, offering a holistic approach that integrates science, nutrition, and the art of flavorful cooking.

At the heart of this guide lies a profound understanding of renal health. The kidneys, those bean-shaped organs nestled within our lower backs, play a pivotal role in maintaining homeostasis within our bodies. From filtering waste products to regulating blood pressure and electrolyte balance, the kidneys silently orchestrate a symphony of physiological processes. The "Renal Reset" concept embodied in this guide represents a call to recalibrate and revitalize these indispensable organs through purposeful nutrition.

The cookbook's genesis stems from a recognition that nourishing the kidneys demands a nuanced and intentional approach to our dietary choices. Every recipe within these pages has been meticulously crafted to cater to the intricate needs of renal health without compromising on the pleasure of eating. It's a culinary journey that transforms the kitchen into a sanctuary where health and taste converge seamlessly.

The cornerstone of this guide is its dedication to providing a diverse array of kidney-friendly recipes. From vibrant salads and soul-satisfying soups to hearty mains and delectable desserts, each dish is a testament to the notion that nourishing our kidneys need not be a mundane or restrictive affair. Instead, it invites us to embrace a world of flavors and textures while keeping a watchful eye on the health of our vital organs.

But this guide goes beyond mere recipes; it is a holistic educational resource. Nestled within its pages are insights into the nutritional intricacies of each ingredient, empowering readers to make informed choices. Understanding the synergy between nutrients and their impact on renal function is the first step toward cultivating a mindful and health-conscious approach to eating.

Navigating this culinary journey, the "Renal Reset" guide places an emphasis on whole, unprocessed foods. It encourages a departure from the pitfalls of modern diets laden with excessive salt, refined sugars, and processed foods — all known adversaries to kidney health. In their stead, the recipes advocate for the incorporation of nutrient-dense, kidney-friendly ingredients that not only support renal function but also contribute to overall well-being.

Moreover, the guide offers practical tips and strategies for meal planning, ensuring that adherence to a kidney-friendly diet is both sustainable and enjoyable. It is a roadmap for individuals seeking to adopt healthier eating habits without sacrificing the joy and fulfillment derived from sharing a delicious meal with loved ones.

As we immerse ourselves in the "Nourishing Dietary Guide for Renal Reset," we become cognizant of the transformative power that intentional nutrition holds. This is not just a cookbook; it is a manifesto for those who seek to take charge of their health, to embark on a journey of renewal, and to savor the richness of life through the prism of kidney-conscious culinary delights.

In conclusion, the "Nourishing Dietary Guide for Renal Reset: Cookbook with Kidney-Friendly Recipes for Optimal Health and Well-being" beckons us to embrace a harmonious approach to nourishment — one that not only tantalizes our taste buds but also honors the silent sentinels of our well-being, our kidneys. It is a celebration of the profound connection between food and health, a testament to the transformative potential that lies within the choices we make in our kitchens every day. So, let the culinary adventure begin, and may it be a journey toward renewed vitality, one delicious recipe at a time.

CHAPTER 1

Understanding Renal Health

Understanding renal health is essential for maintaining overall well-being. The kidneys, two bean-shaped organs located on either side of the spine, play a crucial role in filtering waste products and excess fluids from the blood, regulating electrolyte balance, and producing hormones that control blood pressure. A comprehensive understanding of renal health encompasses various aspects, from anatomy and function to common disorders, prevention, and lifestyle choices.

The kidneys are marvels of biological engineering, consisting of millions of nephrons, the functional units responsible for filtering blood. Each nephron filters blood, removes waste, and reabsorbs essential substances, ensuring a delicate balance. The filtration process involves the glomerulus, a network of tiny blood vessels, and the renal tubules, where the actual filtration and reabsorption occur. This intricate system allows the kidneys to maintain a stable internal environment.

The kidneys' primary function is waste elimination. They filter out toxins, excess salts, and fluids, producing urine as the byproduct. This process helps prevent the buildup of harmful substances in the body, maintaining a healthy balance of electrolytes and preventing conditions like electrolyte imbalances, which can lead to complications such as muscle cramps, weakness, or even cardiac arrhythmias.

Renal health is closely tied to blood pressure regulation. The kidneys release renin, an enzyme that plays a pivotal role in maintaining blood pressure by influencing blood vessel constriction. Imbalances in this mechanism can result in hypertension, a leading cause of kidney disease. Chronic kidney disease (CKD) is a progressive condition that can be caused by hypertension, diabetes, or other underlying conditions. It's crucial to monitor blood pressure regularly and manage it effectively to preserve renal health.

Diabetes, a widespread metabolic disorder, poses a significant threat to renal health. Persistent high blood sugar levels can damage the blood vessels in the kidneys, leading to diabetic nephropathy. This condition progresses slowly, often unnoticed until advanced stages. Regular monitoring of blood glucose levels and early intervention are crucial in preventing diabetic nephropathy and preserving renal function.

Kidney stones, another common renal issue, can cause excruciating pain. These hard deposits form when minerals and salts crystallize in the urine. Dehydration, dietary factors, and genetics contribute to stone formation. Increasing fluid intake, adopting a balanced diet, and managing underlying conditions can aid in preventing kidney stones.

Maintaining optimal renal health extends beyond medical interventions. Lifestyle choices, including a balanced diet, regular exercise, and avoiding excessive alcohol and tobacco consumption, play a crucial role. A diet rich in fruits, vegetables, and whole grains provides essential nutrients and antioxidants that support renal function. Exercise promotes cardiovascular health, reducing the risk of hypertension and related kidney issues.

Hydration is paramount for kidney health. A well-hydrated body supports efficient filtration and prevents the concentration of urine, reducing the risk of kidney stones. Adequate fluid intake also aids in flushing out toxins and promoting overall urinary tract health.

Regular check-ups and screenings are vital for early detection of renal issues. Monitoring kidney function through blood tests, urine analysis, and imaging studies allows healthcare professionals to identify problems in their early stages when interventions can be more effective. Individuals with a family history of kidney disease or those with pre-existing conditions like diabetes should be especially vigilant.

In conclusion, understanding renal health involves grasping the intricate workings of the kidneys, recognizing common disorders, and adopting a holistic approach to prevention and maintenance. By prioritizing lifestyle choices, monitoring blood pressure and blood sugar levels, and seeking timely medical attention, individuals can safeguard their kidneys and promote long-term renal health.

Importance of Kidney-Friendly Diet

A kidney-friendly diet plays a pivotal role in maintaining overall health and preventing the progression of kidney disease. As the body's natural filtration system, kidneys are responsible for removing waste and excess fluids, balancing electrolytes, and regulating blood pressure. Therefore, adopting a diet that supports kidney function is crucial for those with existing kidney issues or those aiming to prevent such complications.

One of the fundamental aspects of a kidney-friendly diet is managing protein intake. Proteins are essential for body functions, but when kidneys are compromised, excessive protein consumption can strain these vital organs. Choosing high-quality, plant-based proteins like legumes, tofu, and grains over animal proteins can help maintain a balance without overburdening the kidneys.

Sodium, a common component of many processed foods, is another factor to consider. Excessive sodium intake can lead to high blood pressure, putting additional strain on the kidneys. A kidney-friendly diet emphasizes low-sodium alternatives, encouraging individuals to choose fresh fruits and vegetables, and opt for herbs and spices for flavoring instead of salt.

Fluid intake is intricately linked to kidney health. While staying hydrated is important, those with kidney issues may need to monitor their fluid intake more closely. Proper hydration supports kidney function but excessive fluids can strain compromised kidneys. Striking the right balance is key, and individual requirements may vary based on the severity of kidney disease and other health factors.

Potassium is an electrolyte that plays a vital role in maintaining proper muscle and nerve function, but imbalances can pose risks, especially for individuals with kidney problems. A kidney-friendly diet provides guidelines for managing potassium intake by moderating the consumption of high-potassium foods like bananas, oranges, and tomatoes.

Phosphorus is another mineral that needs attention in a kidney-friendly diet. Excessive phosphorus can lead to bone and heart complications, common in advanced kidney disease. Restricting phosphorus-rich foods, such as dairy products and certain processed foods, is a key component of managing kidney health through diet.

Furthermore, maintaining a healthy weight is crucial for kidney function. Obesity is linked to an increased risk of kidney disease and can exacerbate existing conditions. A kidney-friendly diet focuses on balanced, nutrient-dense meals that support overall well-being and weight management.

The impact of a kidney-friendly diet extends beyond the physiological realm, influencing mental and emotional well-being. Individuals diagnosed with kidney disease often face dietary restrictions that can be challenging to navigate. A well-structured kidney-friendly diet not only addresses the physical aspects but also provides a sense of control and empowerment over one's health, fostering a positive mindset.

Social support is integral to successfully implementing a kidney-friendly diet. Engaging with support groups, healthcare professionals, and nutritionists can offer guidance, share experiences, and provide practical tips for incorporating dietary changes into daily life. This communal approach helps individuals facing kidney challenges feel less isolated and more equipped to manage their health effectively.

In conclusion, the importance of a kidney-friendly diet cannot be overstated. It is a multifaceted approach that involves mindful choices related to protein, sodium, fluid, potassium, and phosphorus intake. Beyond the physiological benefits, a kidney-friendly diet contributes to mental and emotional well-being, offering a holistic approach to managing kidney health. With the right dietary adjustments, individuals can enhance their quality of life, slow the progression of kidney disease, and reduce the risk of complications associated with impaired kidney function.

CHAPTER 2

Basics of Renal Nutrition

Proper renal nutrition is crucial for maintaining kidney health and managing various renal conditions. The kidneys play a vital role in filtering waste products and excess fluids from the blood, and a balanced diet is essential to support their function. Understanding the basics of renal nutrition involves recognizing dietary components that can impact kidney health, making informed food choices, and managing nutrient intake to promote overall well-being.

One fundamental aspect of renal nutrition is controlling the intake of protein. Protein is an essential nutrient that provides the body with amino acids necessary for various functions, but excessive protein consumption can strain the kidneys. Individuals with renal issues, such as chronic kidney disease (CKD), often need to limit their protein intake to reduce the kidneys' workload. This limitation aims to prevent the accumulation of waste products resulting from

protein metabolism. Choosing high-quality protein sources, such as lean meats, poultry, fish, eggs, and dairy, can help meet nutritional needs while managing protein intake.

Sodium, another key component in renal nutrition, plays a crucial role in fluid balance. Excessive sodium intake can lead to fluid retention and increased blood pressure, placing additional stress on the kidneys. Individuals with kidney conditions are commonly advised to limit their sodium intake. This involves reducing the consumption of processed and packaged foods, which are often high in sodium, and opting for fresh, whole foods. Herbs and spices can be used to enhance flavor without relying on salt, promoting a kidney-friendly diet.

Controlling phosphorus intake is essential for those with impaired kidney function. Phosphorus is a mineral found in many foods, and its balance is disrupted in individuals with CKD. Elevated phosphorus levels can lead to complications such as bone problems and cardiovascular issues. Restricting phosphorus often involves avoiding high-phosphorus foods, including certain dairy products, nuts, seeds, and processed foods containing phosphate additives. Additionally, individuals may be prescribed phosphorus binders to help control phosphorus absorption from the digestive tract.

Potassium is another electrolyte that requires attention in renal nutrition. The kidneys play a significant role in regulating potassium levels, and imbalances can have adverse effects on heart function. In renal conditions, potassium retention can occur, necessitating dietary adjustments. Foods rich in potassium, such as bananas, oranges, potatoes, and tomatoes, may need to be limited. However, individual potassium needs vary, and dietary restrictions should be personalized based on blood test results and medical advice.

Fluid management is a critical aspect of renal nutrition. Proper hydration is essential for overall health, but individuals with kidney issues may need to monitor their fluid intake. Fluid restrictions may be necessary for those with advanced kidney disease to prevent fluid buildup in the body. Monitoring thirst and adjusting fluid intake based on individual needs and medical recommendations is crucial for maintaining hydration while managing renal conditions.

Carbohydrates are a primary energy source in the diet, and their consumption is generally encouraged. However, individuals with diabetes, a common comorbidity in renal conditions, need to manage their carbohydrate intake to control blood sugar levels. Maintaining stable blood sugar levels is important for preventing further kidney damage and managing overall health. Choosing complex carbohydrates, such as whole grains, legumes, and vegetables, can provide sustained energy without causing rapid spikes in blood sugar.

Vitamins and minerals play various roles in overall health, and their significance is heightened for individuals with renal conditions. While a well-balanced diet typically provides essential nutrients, those with impaired kidney function may require specific supplements. For example, individuals with CKD may need vitamin D supplementation, as the kidneys play a role in converting vitamin D into its active form. Regular monitoring of vitamin and mineral levels through blood tests helps ensure adequate supplementation while preventing excess, which can be harmful.

In conclusion, renal nutrition is a nuanced and vital aspect of managing kidney health. Understanding the basics involves navigating the complexities of protein, sodium, phosphorus, potassium, fluid, carbohydrates, and micronutrients. Personalized dietary plans, often developed in collaboration with healthcare professionals and dietitians, are crucial for individuals with renal conditions. By making informed food choices and managing nutrient intake, individuals can support kidney function, prevent complications, and enhance overall well-bein

Nutritional Requirements for Kidney Health

Proper nutrition plays a crucial role in maintaining kidney health, as the kidneys are vital organs responsible for filtering waste products and excess fluids from the blood. Various dietary factors can impact kidney function, and understanding the nutritional requirements for kidney health is essential for preventing complications and supporting overall well-being.

1. Fluid Intake:
 Adequate hydration is fundamental for kidney health. Water helps in the elimination of waste products through urine and prevents the formation of kidney stones. However, individuals with kidney issues may need to manage their fluid intake carefully, as excessive fluid can strain the kidneys. Consulting with a healthcare professional to determine the appropriate amount of daily fluid intake is advisable.

2. Protein Intake:
 Protein is essential for the body's growth and repair, but excessive protein intake can burden the kidneys. Individuals with kidney disease may need to moderate their protein consumption, especially animal proteins. Plant-based protein sources like

beans, lentils, and tofu can be healthier alternatives, as they are generally lower in phosphorus, a mineral that needs to be controlled in kidney disease.

3. Sodium Control:
High sodium intake can lead to elevated blood pressure and fluid retention, placing additional stress on the kidneys. Monitoring and reducing sodium intake by avoiding processed foods, canned soups, and excess salt during cooking can help manage blood pressure and support kidney health.

4. Phosphorus and Potassium Management:
Kidney patients often need to regulate phosphorus and potassium levels in their diet. High levels of these minerals can be harmful to individuals with compromised kidney function. Foods rich in phosphorus, such as dairy products and nuts, should be consumed in moderation. Similarly, potassium-rich foods like bananas and oranges may need to be limited. A dietitian can provide personalized guidance on managing these mineral levels.

5. Calcium Balance:
Maintaining a proper balance of calcium is crucial for kidney health. Individuals with kidney disease may experience issues with calcium absorption,

leading to bone problems. Adequate calcium intake, along with vitamin D, is essential to support bone health. Again, consulting with a healthcare professional or dietitian can help tailor calcium intake based on individual needs.

6. Limiting Oxalate-Rich Foods:
 Oxalates can have a role in the production of kidney stones. Foods high in oxalates, such as beets, chocolate, and certain nuts, may need to be limited in the diet. However, complete avoidance is not necessary, and moderation is key to preventing kidney stone formation.

7. Maintaining a Healthy Weight:
 Obesity is a risk factor for kidney disease. Adopting a balanced diet and engaging in regular physical activity can help maintain a healthy weight and reduce the risk of kidney-related complications.

8. Monitoring Blood Sugar Levels:
 High blood sugar levels can wreak havoc on the kidneys.For individuals with diabetes, managing blood sugar levels through diet, medication, and lifestyle modifications is crucial in preventing kidney complications.

9. Vitamin and Mineral Supplementation:
In some cases, individuals with kidney disease may require vitamin and mineral supplements to address deficiencies. However, supplementation should be approached cautiously, as excessive intake can have adverse effects. Healthcare professionals can determine specific needs and recommend appropriate supplements.

10. Regular Monitoring and Consultation:
Regular check-ups with healthcare providers and consultations with dietitians are essential for individuals with kidney disease. Monitoring blood tests, such as creatinine and glomerular filtration rate (GFR), helps assess kidney function and guides adjustments to the dietary plan.

In conclusion, maintaining optimal kidney health involves a combination of mindful dietary choices, fluid management, and lifestyle modifications. Individualized guidance from healthcare professionals and dietitians is crucial to tailor nutritional recommendations based on the specific needs and health status of each person. By adopting a holistic approach to kidney health, individuals can reduce the risk of complications and promote overall well-being.

Key Nutrients and Their Role

Proper kidney function is essential for maintaining overall health, and a balanced intake of key nutrients plays a pivotal role in supporting these vital organs. The kidneys, two bean-shaped organs located on either side of the spine, are responsible for filtering blood, removing waste products, and regulating fluid balance. Various nutrients contribute to kidney health, supporting their functions and preventing potential complications.

1. Water: The Foundation of Kidney Health
Water is the fundamental nutrient for kidney health. Adequate hydration is crucial for maintaining optimal blood flow to the kidneys, ensuring efficient filtration and waste elimination. Insufficient water intake can lead to the formation of kidney stones and hinder the kidneys' ability to remove toxins.

2. Electrolytes: Balancing Act
Electrolytes, including sodium, potassium, and chloride, play a crucial role in maintaining the balance of fluids in and around cells. Proper electrolyte balance is essential for kidney function, as these minerals help regulate blood pressure and facilitate nerve impulses. An imbalance can lead to hypertension and negatively impact kidney health.
3. Protein: Building Blocks and Caution

Protein is necessary for the body's general operation and tissue repair. However, excessive protein intake can strain the kidneys. It is important to strike a balance, ensuring an adequate but not excessive amount of protein to prevent kidney damage. High-quality sources, such as lean meats, fish, and legumes, are preferable for kidney health.

4. Vitamins: Antioxidant Defense
Vitamins, particularly antioxidants like vitamin C and E, contribute to kidney health by neutralizing harmful free radicals. Free radicals can damage cells, including those in the kidneys, and antioxidants help protect against this oxidative stress. Fruits, vegetables, and nuts are rich sources of these vital vitamins.
5. Minerals: The Role of Calcium and Phosphorus
Calcium and phosphorus are minerals that play a crucial role in bone health, and their balance is essential for kidney function. Abnormal levels of these minerals can contribute to the formation of kidney stones. Maintaining an appropriate ratio of calcium to phosphorus in the diet, along with adequate vitamin D, helps support both bone and kidney health.

6. Omega-3 Fatty Acids: Inflammation Control
Omega-3 fatty acids, found in fatty fish like salmon and flaxseeds, possess anti-inflammatory properties that can benefit kidney health. Chronic inflammation is associated with kidney disease, and incorporating omega-3-rich foods into the diet may help mitigate inflammation and reduce the risk of kidney damage.

7. Fiber: Digestive Health
A diet rich in fiber promotes digestive health and helps manage blood sugar levels. High-fiber foods, including whole grains, fruits, and vegetables, contribute to overall well-being and may indirectly support kidney health by reducing the risk of conditions like diabetes, which can negatively impact kidney function.

8. Magnesium: Maintaining Balance
Magnesium is involved in various biochemical reactions in the body, including those related to kidney function. It helps regulate blood pressure and supports muscle and nerve function. Consuming magnesium-rich foods like nuts, seeds, and leafy greens contributes to maintaining a balance that supports kidney health.

9. Limiting Sodium: Managing Blood Pressure
Excessive sodium intake can contribute to high blood pressure, putting a strain on the kidneys. Limiting sodium in the diet is crucial for

maintaining healthy blood pressure levels and reducing the risk of kidney damage. Reading food labels and choosing low-sodium options can aid in achieving this balance.

In conclusion, a well-rounded and balanced diet, along with proper hydration, is integral to supporting kidney health. Each nutrient plays a unique role, from maintaining fluid balance to combating inflammation and oxidative stress. Striking the right balance and being mindful of the quality and quantity of nutrients consumed can go a long way in promoting optimal kidney function and preventing potential complications. As always, consulting with a healthcare professional or a registered dietitian for personalized advice is recommended, especially for individuals with pre-existing kidney conditions or specific dietary needs.

CHAPTER 3

Renal Reset Principles

Renal Reset Principles refer to a set of guidelines and practices aimed at optimizing renal (kidney) function and promoting overall kidney health. The kidneys play a crucial role in maintaining the body's internal environment by filtering blood, removing waste products, and regulating fluid and electrolyte balance. Adhering to Renal Reset Principles involves adopting lifestyle changes, dietary adjustments, and maintaining proper hydration to support optimal kidney function. Here, we'll explore key aspects of Renal Reset Principles in detail.

1. Hydration:

One fundamental principle of renal health is adequate hydration. Proper fluid intake ensures that the kidneys can effectively filter waste products from the blood and maintain electrolyte balance. Water is the best choice for hydration, and individuals should aim to drink enough water throughout the day. However, excessive water intake should be avoided, as it can put unnecessary strain on the kidneys.

2. Balanced Diet:

A well-balanced diet is essential for renal health. Renal Reset Principles emphasize the importance of consuming a variety of nutrient-dense foods, including fruits, vegetables, whole grains, and lean proteins. Monitoring salt intake is crucial, as excessive salt can contribute to high blood pressure and kidney damage. Additionally, limiting the consumption of processed foods, which often contain high levels of sodium, is advisable.

3. Monitoring Protein Intake:

Although an excessive protein diet might cause renal strain, protein is necessary for good health overall.Renal Reset Principles recommend monitoring and moderating protein consumption, especially for individuals with existing kidney conditions. High-quality protein sources, such as lean meats, fish, and plant-based proteins, are preferred over processed or red meats.

4. Blood Pressure Management:

Controlling blood pressure is a key aspect of Renal Reset Principles. Hypertension can damage the small blood vessels in the kidneys, impairing their function over time. Lifestyle modifications, including regular exercise, a low-sodium diet, and stress management, contribute to maintaining healthy blood pressure levels.

5. Regular Physical Activity:
Exercise is beneficial for overall health,
including renal health. Regular physical activity
helps regulate blood pressure, manage weight,
and improve cardiovascular function, all of
which indirectly support kidney function. Renal
Reset Principles encourage incorporating
moderate exercise into daily routines.

6. Avoiding Nephrotoxic Substances:
Certain substances can be harmful to the
kidneys. Renal Reset Principles advise against
the excessive use of over-the-counter pain
medications, non-steroidal anti-inflammatory
drugs (NSAIDs), and other nephrotoxic
substances. These can contribute to kidney
damage, particularly if used over extended
periods or in high doses.

7. Regular Monitoring and Check-ups:
Routine health check-ups and monitoring
kidney function through blood tests are integral
to Renal Reset Principles. Early detection of
any abnormalities allows for timely intervention
and can prevent the progression of kidney
disease. Individuals with a family history of
kidney problems or those with pre-existing
conditions should be particularly vigilant.

8. Managing Diabetes:
Diabetes is a leading cause of kidney disease.
Renal Reset Principles stress the importance
of managing blood sugar levels through a
combination of medication, a balanced diet,
and regular monitoring. Controlling diabetes
effectively can significantly reduce the risk of
kidney complications.

9. Smoking Cessation:
Smoking has detrimental effects on the
cardiovascular system, including blood vessels
in the kidneys. Renal Reset Principles
advocate for smoking cessation to reduce the
risk of kidney damage and support overall
cardiovascular health.

10. Stress Reduction:
Prolonged stress can have a detrimental effect
on renal function as well as general
health.Renal Reset Principles include stress
reduction strategies such as mindfulness,
meditation, and other relaxation techniques to
promote mental and physical well-being.

In conclusion, Renal Reset Principles
encompass a holistic approach to kidney
health, incorporating hydration, a balanced
diet, regular exercise, blood pressure
management, and various lifestyle
adjustments. By adhering to these principles,

individuals can proactively support their renal function, reduce the risk of kidney disease, and enhance overall well-being. It is important to note that these principles are general guidelines, and individuals with specific medical conditions should consult healthcare professionals for personalized advice.

Resetting Your Diet for Kidney Wellness

Resetting your diet for kidney wellness is a transformative journey that involves making mindful choices to support the health of these vital organs. The kidneys play a crucial role in filtering waste and excess fluids from the blood, maintaining electrolyte balance, and regulating blood pressure. Adopting a kidney-friendly diet can contribute significantly to their well-being and overall health. In this exploration, we'll delve into the principles of a kidney-friendly diet, the foods to embrace and avoid, and the impact of lifestyle choices on renal health.

Understanding the Basics

The foundation of a kidney-friendly diet lies in managing key nutrients, particularly sodium, potassium, and phosphorus. Monitoring these elements helps maintain a balance that supports kidney function without overburdening them. It's crucial to work closely with healthcare professionals and dieticians to tailor dietary recommendations to individual needs, as kidney conditions can vary.

1. Sodium Sensibility

Reducing sodium intake is a cornerstone of kidney wellness. High sodium levels can lead to increased blood pressure, putting extra strain on the kidneys. Opting for fresh, whole foods over processed alternatives can significantly cut down on sodium intake. Flavoring dishes with herbs and spices instead of salt is a flavorful alternative that promotes kidney health.

2. Potassium Paradox

While potassium is an essential nutrient for many bodily functions, kidney patients often need to manage their potassium levels. Foods high in potassium, such as potatoes, bananas, and oranges, should be eaten in moderation.Striking a balance is key, ensuring adequate potassium for health without overwhelming compromised kidneys.

3. Phosphorus Puzzle

Phosphorus, another critical mineral, can accumulate in the bloodstream when kidneys are impaired. Dairy products, nuts, and seeds are high in phosphorus, and limiting their intake is essential. Understanding food labels is crucial, as hidden phosphorus in processed foods can catch one off guard.

Embracing Kidney-Friendly Foods

1. Vegetable Variety

Incorporating a rainbow of vegetables into the diet provides a plethora of nutrients without overloading on problematic minerals. Leafy greens, bell peppers, and cabbage are excellent choices. These not only add nutritional value but also contribute to overall well-being.

2. Lean Protein Practices

Protein is a vital component, but excessive protein consumption can strain the kidneys. Opting for lean sources like poultry, fish, and tofu ensures a balance that supports muscle health without overtaxing the kidneys. Portion control is key in maintaining this delicate equilibrium.

3. Hydration Habits

Adequate hydration is paramount for kidney health.Water aids in the removal of pollutants and stops kidney stones from forming. Monitoring fluid intake is essential, especially for individuals with fluid retention concerns.

Striking a balance between staying hydrated and managing fluid retention is a delicate but crucial task.

Avoiding Kidney Culprits

1. Processed Perils

Processed foods often harbor hidden sodium, phosphorus, and potassium. Steering clear of these items minimizes the risk of inadvertently compromising kidney health. Opting for whole, unprocessed foods ensures better control over nutrient intake.

2. Sugary Snares

Excessive sugar intake can contribute to diabetes and obesity, both of which are risk factors for kidney disease. Choosing natural sweeteners or moderating sugar consumption supports overall health and aids in kidney wellness.

3. Caffeine Caution

While moderate caffeine consumption is generally considered safe, excessive intake can lead to dehydration, potentially impacting kidney function. Maintaining a balanced approach to caffeine, including sources like tea

and limiting sugary caffeinated beverages, is
wise.

Lifestyle and Kidney Harmony

1. Exercise Elegance

Kidney function is one aspect of overall health
that is supported by regular physical
exercise.Exercise helps manage weight, blood
pressure, and reduces the risk of chronic
conditions that can compromise renal health.
Tailoring an exercise routine to individual
needs and consulting healthcare professionals
ensures a safe and effective approach.

2. Stress Relief Strategies

Chronic stress can contribute to various health
issues, including kidney problems.
Incorporating stress-relief practices such as
meditation, yoga, or mindfulness into daily life
promotes not only mental well-being but also
supports overall kidney health.

3. Regular Monitoring

For individuals with existing kidney conditions,
regular monitoring through blood tests and
check-ups is essential. This proactive

approach allows for timely adjustments to dietary and lifestyle choices, ensuring that the kidneys are well-supported.

In conclusion, resetting your diet for kidney wellness is a multifaceted journey that encompasses dietary choices, lifestyle adjustments, and regular monitoring. By understanding the nuances of a kidney-friendly diet, embracing wholesome foods, and making mindful lifestyle choices, individuals can actively contribute to the well-being of their kidneys. It's a journey of empowerment and self-care, guided by the principles of balance and moderation, ultimately paving the way for a healthier, more vibrant life.

Lifestyle Changes for Optimal Renal Health

Maintaining optimal renal health is crucial for overall well-being, and lifestyle changes play a pivotal role in achieving and sustaining it. The kidneys, often overlooked, are intricate organs responsible for filtering waste from the blood, regulating fluid balance, and supporting various bodily functions. Incorporating healthy habits into one's lifestyle can significantly impact renal health positively.

Dietary Choices:
A fundamental aspect of promoting optimal renal health lies in mindful dietary choices. A diet low in sodium helps control blood pressure, reducing the strain on the kidneys. Additionally, limiting phosphorus-rich foods is essential for those with kidney issues. Embracing a plant-based diet with ample fruits and vegetables provides essential vitamins and antioxidants while naturally lowering the intake of potentially harmful substances.

Hydration is Key:
Adequate hydration is crucial for kidney function. Water helps flush toxins from the body and prevents the formation of kidney stones. Individuals should aim to consume a

sufficient amount of water throughout the day, and this becomes especially important during warmer weather or physical activity.

Regular Exercise:
Engaging in regular physical activity contributes to overall health and aids in maintaining optimal renal function. Exercise helps control weight, regulate blood pressure, and improve cardiovascular health – all factors that indirectly benefit the kidneys. However, it's crucial to strike a balance, as excessive strenuous exercise can potentially harm kidney health.

Maintaining Healthy Blood Pressure:
Kidney injury is mostly caused by high blood pressure. Lifestyle changes such as reducing salt intake, regular exercise, and stress management can contribute to maintaining healthy blood pressure levels. Regular monitoring of blood pressure is imperative, and any deviations from the norm should be promptly addressed with healthcare professionals.

Quit Smoking and Limit Alcohol Intake:
Smoking and excessive alcohol consumption have detrimental effects on kidney health. Smoking reduces blood flow to the kidneys, impairing their function, while alcohol can lead to dehydration and negatively impact blood

pressure. Quitting smoking and moderating alcohol intake are pivotal steps towards optimal renal health.

Manage Chronic Conditions:
Chronic conditions like diabetes and hypertension significantly increase the risk of kidney disease. Effectively managing these conditions through medication, lifestyle changes, and regular medical check-ups is vital. Consistent monitoring and control of blood sugar levels help prevent diabetic nephropathy, a severe complication affecting the kidneys.

Maintain a Healthy Weight:
Obesity is a risk factor for kidney disease. Adopting a healthy and balanced diet, combined with regular physical activity, aids in weight management. Weight loss can alleviate stress on the kidneys and reduce the likelihood of developing kidney-related complications.

Adequate Sleep:
Quality sleep is often underestimated but plays a crucial role in overall health, including renal health. Chronic sleep deprivation can contribute to conditions like hypertension and diabetes, both of which have a direct impact on kidney function. Prioritizing a good night's sleep is a simple yet effective lifestyle change.

Stress Management:
Chronic stress has been linked to renal damage among other health problems.Incorporating stress-reduction techniques such as meditation, yoga, or deep breathing exercises into daily routines can promote mental well-being and indirectly support optimal renal health.

Regular Health Check-ups:
Regular medical check-ups enable early detection and intervention in case of any emerging renal issues. Routine blood pressure monitoring, kidney function tests, and urine tests can provide valuable insights into the health of these vital organs. Early detection allows for timely intervention and management, preventing the progression of potential kidney problems.

In conclusion, lifestyle changes are pivotal in promoting optimal renal health. Adopting a holistic approach that includes a balanced diet, hydration, regular exercise, and stress management can significantly reduce the risk of kidney disease. These changes not only benefit the kidneys but contribute to overall well-being, emphasizing the interconnectedness of lifestyle and health. Making informed choices and embracing a kidney-friendly lifestyle is an investment in long-term health and vitality.

CHAPTER 4

Kidney-Friendly Foods

Kidney-friendly foods play a crucial role in maintaining the health of individuals with kidney issues. The kidneys are vital organs responsible for filtering waste products and excess fluids from the blood, helping to regulate blood pressure and electrolyte balance. When kidney function is compromised, it becomes essential to adopt a diet that supports renal health. This article will explore various kidney-friendly foods, their benefits, and tips for maintaining a balanced and nutritious diet for individuals with kidney concerns.

1. Low-Potassium Fruits:
- Incorporating fruits with low potassium content is crucial for kidney health. Examples include apples, berries, and grapes. These fruits provide essential vitamins and antioxidants without overloading the body with potassium, which can be challenging for compromised kidneys to process.

2. Vegetables:
- Vegetables such as cauliflower, bell peppers, and cabbage are low in potassium and are excellent choices for kidney-friendly diets. These vegetables offer fiber, vitamins, and minerals without burdening the kidneys.

3. Lean Proteins:

 - High-quality, lean protein sources like chicken, fish, and eggs are essential for individuals with kidney issues. These proteins provide necessary amino acids without contributing to excessive waste products that the kidneys must filter.

4. Grains and Starches:

 - Opting for whole grains like brown rice and quinoa over refined grains supports a kidney-friendly diet. These grains are rich in fiber and nutrients without causing spikes in blood sugar or contributing to excessive phosphorus intake.

5. Healthy Fats:

 - Incorporating sources of healthy fats, such as olive oil and avocados, can benefit kidney health. These fats provide essential fatty acids and contribute to overall cardiovascular health, which is often interconnected with kidney function.

6. Low-Sodium Choices:

 - Monitoring sodium intake is crucial for individuals with kidney concerns, as excess sodium can lead to fluid retention and increased blood pressure. Choosing low-sodium alternatives and minimizing processed foods can help maintain a kidney-friendly diet.

7. Berries:
 - Berries, including strawberries, blueberries, and raspberries, are not only low in potassium but also packed with antioxidants. Antioxidants play a role in reducing inflammation and oxidative stress, which can be beneficial for kidney health.

8. Red Bell Peppers:
 - Red bell peppers are a great source of vitamins A, C, and B6, as well as fiber. They are low in potassium and can be a flavorful addition to various dishes, providing essential nutrients without compromising kidney health.

9. Cabbage:
 - Cabbage is a low-potassium vegetable that can be included in a kidney-friendly diet. It offers vitamins, minerals, and phytonutrients while being gentle on the kidneys.

10. Apples:
 - Apples are a kidney-friendly fruit that provides fiber and various vitamins without contributing excessive potassium. The soluble fiber in apples may also help with digestion and overall gut health.

Tips for a Kidney-Friendly Diet:

Fluid Intake: Adequate fluid intake is essential, but the amount may vary based on individual needs. Consultation with a healthcare professional can help determine the appropriate fluid intake for each person.

Phosphorus Control: Monitoring phosphorus intake is crucial, as elevated phosphorus levels can be harmful to kidney function. Limiting the consumption of phosphorus-rich foods like dairy products and processed foods is advisable.

Portion Control: Controlling portion sizes helps manage nutrient intake and reduces the workload on the kidneys. Smaller, more frequent meals can be easier for the kidneys to process.

Consultation with a Dietitian: Individuals with kidney concerns should consult with a registered dietitian or healthcare professional to create a personalized and effective kidney-friendly diet plan.

In conclusion, adopting a kidney-friendly diet is essential for individuals with compromised kidney function. Emphasizing low-potassium fruits, vegetables, lean proteins, and healthy fats while monitoring sodium and phosphorus intake can contribute to overall renal health. Additionally, staying hydrated and seeking guidance from healthcare professionals or dietitians ensures that dietary choices align with individual needs. By making informed and conscious food choices, individuals can better manage their kidney health and enhance their overall well-being.

Incorporating fresh produce

Incorporating fresh produce into renal nutrition is a vital aspect of promoting kidney health and overall well-being for individuals with kidney-related issues. The kidneys play a crucial role in filtering waste and excess fluids from the blood, and maintaining a balanced diet, including an emphasis on fresh produce, is essential to support kidney function. This article explores the benefits of incorporating fresh fruits and vegetables into renal diets, the specific considerations for individuals with renal issues, and practical tips for achieving a kidney-friendly, plant-based nutrition plan.

Benefits of Fresh Produce in Renal Nutrition

1. Nutrient-Rich Content:
Fresh produce, including fruits and vegetables, is rich in essential nutrients such as vitamins, minerals, and antioxidants. These nutrients contribute to overall health and help combat inflammation, a factor that can exacerbate kidney problems.

2. Lower Potassium Content:
Renal diets often require careful management of potassium intake. Fresh produce tends to have lower potassium levels compared to processed foods, making it easier for individuals with kidney issues to control their potassium intake.

3. High Fiber Content:
Fiber is crucial for digestive health and can aid in managing blood sugar levels. Many fruits and vegetables are excellent sources of dietary fiber, promoting digestive regularity and supporting glycemic control.

4. Hydration Support:
Some fresh produce, like watermelon and cucumber, has high water content, contributing to hydration. Adequate hydration is essential for kidney function, as it helps flush out toxins and waste products from the body.

5. Heart Health Benefits:
Renal patients often face an increased risk of cardiovascular issues. Fresh produce, with its low sodium and high potassium content, can contribute to better blood pressure management and overall heart health.

Considerations for Renal Diets

1. Potassium Control:
While fresh produce is generally lower in potassium, individuals with kidney issues must still be mindful of their potassium intake. Working closely with a healthcare professional or dietitian to create a personalized plan is essential to avoid overconsumption.

2. Phosphorus Management:
Some plant-based foods contain phosphorus, which needs to be limited in renal diets. Understanding the phosphorus content of various fruits and vegetables is crucial for individuals with kidney problems to maintain proper phosphorus balance.

3. Fluid Intake Monitoring:
Renal patients often have restrictions on fluid intake. While fresh produce contributes to hydration, it's important to monitor overall fluid consumption, including beverages, to adhere to prescribed limits.

4. Individualized Approach:
Every individual's nutritional needs and tolerances are unique. Tailoring dietary recommendations based on specific health conditions, medications, and individual responses to certain foods is vital for optimal renal nutrition.

Practical Tips for Incorporating Fresh Produce

1. Diverse Selection:
Encourage a variety of fruits and vegetables to ensure a broad spectrum of nutrients. Different colors often signify distinct nutrient profiles, so incorporating a rainbow of produce can enhance overall nutrition.

2. Cooking Techniques:
Experiment with different cooking methods to make fresh produce more palatable. Steaming, boiling, or baking can be gentler on the kidneys compared to frying or sautéing.

3. Portion Control:
While fresh produce is beneficial, moderation is key. Controlling portion sizes helps manage nutrient intake, particularly for substances like potassium and phosphorus that require careful monitoring.

4. Consultation with Professionals:
Seek guidance from healthcare professionals or registered dietitians who specialize in renal nutrition. They can provide personalized advice, taking into account specific dietary restrictions and health conditions.

5. Mindful Snacking:
 Incorporate fresh fruits and vegetables into snacks. This not only adds nutritional value but also helps in controlling portion sizes throughout the day.

Incorporating fresh produce into renal nutrition is a nuanced but essential aspect of managing kidney-related issues. The benefits of nutrient-rich, low-potassium foods cannot be overstated, and a well-balanced, plant-based diet can contribute significantly to overall health for individuals with kidney concerns. However, the key lies in customization—tailoring dietary plans to the unique needs of each individual. With the guidance of healthcare professionals and a mindful approach to nutrition, individuals with renal issues can embrace the positive impact of fresh produce on their well-being.

Lean Proteins for Renal Support

Lean proteins play a crucial role in renal support, as they provide essential nutrients without putting undue strain on the kidneys. Individuals with renal issues often need to manage their protein intake carefully to prevent further damage to the kidneys while ensuring they receive adequate nutrition. In this discussion, we will delve into the importance of lean proteins for renal support, the types of lean proteins that are beneficial, and practical dietary strategies to incorporate them into a renal-friendly diet.

Importance of Lean Proteins in Renal Support:

Proteins are vital for the body's normal functioning, playing a key role in muscle maintenance, immune system support, and overall cellular health. However, for individuals with kidney problems, excessive protein intake, especially from sources high in saturated fats, can exacerbate kidney damage. Lean proteins, characterized by lower fat content, offer a solution by providing essential amino acids without overloading the kidneys.

Lean proteins aid in preserving muscle mass, a concern for those with renal issues who may experience muscle wasting. Additionally, they contribute to a sense of fullness, helping individuals maintain a healthy weight—a crucial aspect of renal health.

Types of Lean Proteins for Renal Support:

1. Poultry: Skinless chicken and turkey breast are excellent sources of lean protein. They are low in fat and can be prepared in various ways, offering versatility in meal planning.

2. Fish: Fatty fish such as salmon, mackerel, and trout are rich in omega-3 fatty acids, which have anti-inflammatory properties. Opting for grilled or baked fish instead of fried varieties ensures a renal-friendly preparation.

3. **Eggs:** Eggs are a complete protein source, providing all essential amino acids. They are a versatile ingredient that can be included in various renal-friendly dishes.

4. Plant-Based Proteins: Legumes, tofu, and tempeh are plant-based protein sources suitable for renal support. They are low in saturated fats and can be included in a renal diet to diversify protein intake.

5. Lean Cuts of Meat: Lean cuts of beef or pork, such as sirloin or tenderloin, can be included in moderation. Trimming visible fats before cooking reduces the fat content further.

****Dietary Strategies for Incorporating Lean Proteins:****

1. Portion Control: Controlling portion sizes is crucial for individuals with renal issues. Smaller, frequent meals help distribute protein intake throughout the day, reducing the workload on the kidneys.

2. Healthy Cooking Methods: Opting for cooking methods such as grilling, baking, or steaming helps maintain the leanness of protein sources. Avoiding frying minimizes the addition of excess fats.

3. Limiting Phosphorus: Some lean protein sources may contain higher levels of phosphorus, which can be problematic for individuals with kidney issues. Monitoring phosphorus intake and choosing low-phosphorus options can help manage this aspect of the diet.

4. Balanced Diet: Combining lean proteins with a variety of fruits, vegetables, and whole grains ensures a well-rounded and nutritionally balanced diet. This approach provides essential vitamins and minerals without relying solely on protein sources.

5. Consultation with a Dietitian: Individual dietary needs can vary, and consulting with a registered dietitian or healthcare professional is crucial for creating a personalized renal-friendly meal plan. They can provide tailored guidance based on the individual's health status, preferences, and dietary restrictions.

In conclusion, incorporating lean proteins into a renal-friendly diet is essential for individuals with kidney issues. These proteins offer the necessary building blocks for bodily functions without placing excessive strain on the kidneys. By choosing lean protein sources wisely, practicing portion control, and adopting healthy cooking methods, individuals can support their renal health while enjoying a varied and satisfying diet. Consulting with healthcare professionals ensures that dietary choices align with individual health needs and goals.

Smart carbohydrate choices

Smart carbohydrate choices play a crucial role in renal support, as individuals with kidney issues need to manage their diet carefully to maintain optimal health. The kidneys play a vital role in filtering waste products from the blood, and for those with renal concerns, monitoring carbohydrate intake becomes essential. In this context, making intelligent decisions about the types and amounts of carbohydrates consumed can contribute significantly to overall kidney health.

One of the primary considerations for individuals with renal issues is to focus on complex carbohydrates rather than simple sugars. Complex carbohydrates, found in foods like whole grains, vegetables, and legumes, take longer to break down, resulting in a slower release of glucose into the bloodstream. This slow release can help in regulating blood sugar levels, preventing unnecessary strain on the kidneys.

Whole grains, such as brown rice, quinoa, and whole wheat products, stand out as excellent choices for renal support. These grains are rich in fiber, which not only aids in digestion but also helps control blood sugar levels. Fiber can be particularly beneficial for individuals with kidney issues, as it assists in maintaining a healthy weight and managing diabetes – conditions often associated with renal concerns.

Vegetables, especially those low in potassium and phosphorus, are another essential component of a renal-friendly diet. Leafy greens like kale and spinach, as well as cruciferous vegetables such as broccoli and cauliflower, are generally lower in potassium and can be included in a renal diet in moderation. Balancing the intake of these vegetables is crucial, as excessive potassium can be problematic for individuals with compromised kidney function.

Legumes, including beans, lentils, and peas, are not only rich in complex carbohydrates but also provide a good source of protein. This is significant for those with renal issues, as managing protein intake is a key aspect of renal support. Choosing plant-based protein sources over animal proteins can help reduce the load on the kidneys, as plant proteins tend to produce fewer waste products during metabolism.

While managing carbohydrate intake is crucial, paying attention to the glycemic index (GI) of foods is equally important. The GI calculates the rate at which a certain food elevates blood sugar. Foods with a lower GI are preferred for renal support, as they lead to a slower increase in blood glucose. Sweet potatoes, for instance, have a lower GI compared to regular potatoes, making them a smarter carbohydrate choice for individuals with kidney concerns.

In addition to specific food choices, portion control plays a pivotal role in managing carbohydrate intake for renal support. Controlling portion sizes helps regulate calorie intake, which is essential for maintaining a healthy weight – a factor closely linked to kidney health. It is advisable for individuals with renal concerns to work with a healthcare professional or a dietitian to determine appropriate portion sizes based on their specific dietary needs.

Another consideration in smart carbohydrate choices for renal support is the limitation of added sugars. Excessive consumption of added sugars can contribute to weight gain and exacerbate conditions such as diabetes, both of which can impact kidney health. Reading food labels to identify hidden sugars and opting for natural sources of sweetness, such as fruits in moderation, can help in making healthier carbohydrate choices.

Hydration is a critical aspect of renal support, and the type of beverages consumed also contributes to overall carbohydrate intake. Sugary drinks should be avoided, as they not only contribute to excessive calorie intake but can also negatively affect blood sugar levels. Water is the best choice for staying hydrated, and herbal teas without added sugars can be a flavorful alternative.

In conclusion, making smart carbohydrate choices for renal support involves a thoughtful selection of complex carbohydrates, attention to the glycemic index, portion control, and a focus on overall dietary balance. Consulting with healthcare professionals or dietitians can provide personalized guidance based on an individual's specific renal needs. By incorporating these intelligent dietary choices, individuals with kidney concerns can play an active role in supporting their overall health and well-being.

CHAPTER 5

Meal Planning Strategies

Meal planning for renal support is crucial to ensure individuals with kidney issues maintain a well-balanced diet that supports their health. Kidney disease often necessitates dietary adjustments to manage protein, phosphorus, potassium, and sodium intake. Here's a comprehensive guide on meal planning strategies tailored for renal support.

Understanding Renal Diet Basics:

A renal diet restricts the amount of particular nutrients that are consumed in an effort to lessen the strain on the kidneys. Key components include:

1. Protein Management:
- Opt for high-quality protein sources like fish, poultry, eggs, and dairy while moderating intake to prevent excess protein breakdown.

- Consider plant-based protein alternatives such as beans, lentils, and tofu to minimize the strain on kidneys.

2. Phosphorus Control:
- Limit phosphorus-rich foods like dairy, nuts, seeds, and whole grains to prevent complications associated with high phosphorus levels.
- Choose low-phosphorus alternatives and prioritize phosphorus binders as recommended by healthcare professionals.

3. Potassium Moderation:
- Manage potassium by selecting low-potassium fruits and vegetables like apples, berries, and green beans.
- Cooking techniques like leaching can help reduce potassium content in certain foods, such as potatoes.

4. Sodium Restriction:
- Monitor sodium intake to control blood pressure and fluid balance.
- Use herbs, spices, and lemon juice as flavor enhancers instead of salt, and choose fresh foods over processed ones.

Practical Meal Planning Strategies:

1. Consultation with a Dietitian:
 - Seek guidance from a registered dietitian who specializes in renal nutrition to create a personalized meal plan based on individual health needs.

2. Balanced Plate Approach:
 - Divide meals into sections: one-fourth protein, one-fourth grains/starch, and half fruits and vegetables to maintain a balanced nutrient intake.

3. Portion Control:
 - Be mindful of portion sizes to avoid overloading the kidneys. Use measuring cups and food scales for accuracy.

4. Meal Frequency:
 - Opt for smaller, more frequent meals to distribute nutrient intake throughout the day and minimize strain on the kidneys.

5. Fluid Management:
 - Monitor fluid intake, including beverages and foods with high water content. Limiting fluids helps regulate fluid balance and prevent edema.

6. Label Reading:
 - Scrutinize food labels for phosphorus and potassium content. Choose products with lower levels of these minerals.

7. Cooking Techniques:
 - Choose cooking methods that retain nutrients while minimizing the addition of unhealthy elements. Steaming, baking, and grilling are preferable to frying.

8. Menu Variety:
 - Plan a diverse menu to ensure a wide range of nutrients without overloading on any specific mineral. Rotate protein sources and vary fruits and vegetables.

9. Educational Resources:
 - Stay informed about renal-friendly recipes and cooking tips through reputable sources, cookbooks, and online platforms dedicated to renal diets.

Sample Renal-Friendly Meal Plan:

Breakfast:
- Oatmeal with sliced apples and cinnamon (low phosphorus and potassium).
- Scrambled eggs or egg whites (protein source).

Lunch:
- Grilled chicken or tofu salad with mixed greens and low-potassium vegetables.
- Quinoa or rice as a side (controlled portion for starch).

Snack:
- Greek yogurt with strawberries (moderate protein and low phosphorus).

Dinner:
- Baked fish with lemon (lean protein).
- Steamed broccoli and carrots (low in potassium).
- Mashed sweet potatoes (lower potassium than regular potatoes).

Snack:
- Handful of almonds (controlled portion for protein).

Conclusion:

Effective meal planning for renal support involves a combination of knowledge, practical strategies, and ongoing collaboration with healthcare professionals. By prioritizing nutrient balance, portion control, and mindful choices, individuals with kidney concerns can maintain a nourishing and kidney-friendly diet to support their overall health and well-being. Always consult with a healthcare provider or a registered dietitian to tailor the meal plan according to specific health conditions and needs.

Balancing nutrients in each meal

Balancing nutrients in each meal is crucial for maintaining overall health, particularly when focusing on renal wellness. While specific diets like the Renal Reset Diet exist, we'll explore general principles of nutrient balance that can support kidney health without explicitly delving into that particular regimen.

Protein is an essential component of any diet, but for individuals aiming to support renal function, it's vital to choose high-quality, low-phosphorus sources. Lean meats like chicken and turkey, fish, eggs, and plant-based proteins such as legumes and tofu can provide necessary protein without excessive phosphorus intake. Controlling protein portions is also key, as excessive protein consumption can strain the kidneys.

Incorporating a variety of colorful vegetables into meals ensures a rich array of vitamins, minerals, and antioxidants. These nutrients play a vital role in supporting the immune system and reducing inflammation, which is particularly important for individuals with compromised renal function. Leafy greens, bell peppers, carrots, and cauliflower are excellent choices, offering an abundance of vitamins while being relatively low in potassium.

Controlling potassium levels is crucial for individuals with renal concerns. While many fruits and vegetables are high in potassium, opting for those with lower potassium content can help strike a balance. Apples, berries, and cabbage are examples of foods that contribute valuable nutrients without excessively elevated potassium levels.

Sodium management is another critical aspect of renal nutrition. High sodium intake can contribute to hypertension and fluid retention, placing additional strain on the kidneys. Choosing fresh, whole foods over processed options can significantly reduce sodium intake. Herbs and spices can be used to enhance flavor without relying on salt, promoting a kidney-friendly diet.

Whole grains are excellent sources of fiber, which aids digestion and helps regulate blood sugar levels. However, some whole grains, such as whole wheat, can be higher in phosphorus. Opting for grains like quinoa, bulgur, and barley that are lower in phosphorus can be a prudent choice for individuals mindful of renal health.

Incorporating healthy fats, such as those found in avocados, olive oil, and nuts, can contribute to a well-rounded diet. These fats provide essential fatty acids that support overall health without negatively impacting kidney function. Monitoring portion sizes is important, as fats are calorie-dense.

Dairy products are a good source of calcium, but individuals with renal concerns must be cautious due to their phosphorus content. Choosing lower-phosphorus dairy options or exploring alternatives like almond or rice milk can help meet calcium needs without compromising renal health.

Hydration is paramount for kidney function. Water aids in the body's removal of waste materials and poisons.While individual fluid needs vary, maintaining adequate hydration without overloading the kidneys is essential. Monitoring fluid intake becomes particularly important for those with renal challenges, and consulting with a healthcare professional can provide personalized guidance.

In conclusion, balancing nutrients in each meal is a fundamental aspect of supporting renal health. Emphasizing high-quality, low-phosphorus proteins, incorporating a variety of colorful vegetables, managing potassium and sodium intake, choosing suitable grains, incorporating healthy fats, and being mindful of fluid intake are all integral components of a kidney-friendly diet. By adopting these principles, individuals can promote overall well-being and support their renal function without explicitly adhering to a specific renal reset diet.

Portion Control and Renal Health

Portion control plays a pivotal role in maintaining renal health, a connection often underestimated in the realm of dietary practices. The kidneys, vital organs responsible for filtering waste and excess fluids from the blood, are highly sensitive to dietary choices. Understanding the impact of portion control on renal health is crucial for preventing conditions such as chronic kidney disease (CKD) and managing existing kidney-related issues.

In essence, portion control involves managing the amount of food consumed in a single sitting. This practice extends beyond weight management; it significantly influences the nutritional balance crucial for overall health, including renal well-being. Excessive intake of certain nutrients can strain the kidneys, exacerbating existing conditions or contributing to the development of kidney problems.

One primary concern related to portion control and renal health is the regulation of sodium intake. Sodium, commonly found in table salt and processed foods, has a direct impact on blood pressure. High blood pressure, or hypertension, is a leading cause of kidney damage. By controlling portion sizes, individuals can effectively moderate their sodium intake, reducing the strain on the kidneys and minimizing the risk of hypertension-related kidney issues.

Furthermore, portion control plays a key role in managing protein consumption. While protein is essential for various bodily functions, excessive intake can be harmful to individuals with compromised kidney function. In cases of CKD, the kidneys struggle to eliminate protein waste products, leading to a buildup of toxins in the bloodstream. By moderating protein portions, individuals with renal issues can alleviate the burden on their kidneys and slow the progression of kidney disease.

Additionally, the type of carbohydrates consumed is crucial for renal health. Portion control aids in managing the intake of refined carbohydrates, which can contribute to diabetes, a significant risk factor for kidney disease. By monitoring portion sizes and choosing complex carbohydrates over refined ones, individuals can help regulate blood sugar levels, reducing the likelihood of diabetes-related kidney complications.

Fat intake also plays a role in renal health, particularly in the context of portion control. While certain fats are essential for a balanced diet, excessive consumption can contribute to obesity and cardiovascular issues, which in turn impact kidney function. Controlling portion sizes helps maintain a healthy balance of fats, supporting overall cardiovascular and renal well-being.

Focusing on nutrient-dense foods within controlled portions is another aspect of promoting renal health. This approach ensures that the body receives essential vitamins and minerals without overloading the kidneys with unnecessary waste products. Adequate portions of fruits, vegetables, and whole grains contribute to a well-rounded diet that supports overall health, including renal function.

Beyond the physiological aspects, portion control also influences lifestyle factors that contribute to renal health. Overeating and obesity are linked to an increased risk of kidney disease. By adopting portion control practices, individuals can manage their weight, reducing the strain on the kidneys and decreasing the likelihood of developing kidney-related complications.

In the context of renal health, hydration is a critical consideration. Proper fluid balance is essential for kidney function, and portion control extends to the regulation of fluid intake. Monitoring fluid consumption is particularly crucial for individuals with kidney issues, as excessive fluid intake can strain the kidneys and lead to complications.

Educating individuals on portion control and its impact on renal health is essential for preventing and managing kidney-related conditions. Healthcare professionals play a vital role in providing guidance on appropriate portion sizes, considering the specific dietary needs of individuals with renal issues. Dietary counseling that emphasizes portion control empowers individuals to make informed choices that support their overall health and well-being.

In conclusion, portion control is a fundamental aspect of maintaining renal health. It influences the intake of key nutrients such as sodium, protein, carbohydrates, and fats, all of which play a significant role in kidney function. By practicing portion control, individuals can reduce the risk of hypertension, diabetes, and obesity, factors that contribute to kidney disease. Embracing a balanced and mindful approach to eating not only benefits overall health but also serves as a proactive measure in preserving renal function and preventing the onset or progression of kidney-related conditions.

CHAPTER 6

Renal Reset Cookbook

The Renal Reset Cookbook is a comprehensive guide designed to support individuals with kidney-related issues in managing their diet and promoting kidney health. With an emphasis on recipes that are low in sodium, potassium, and phosphorus, this cookbook aims to provide delicious and nutritious meals tailored to the specific dietary needs of those with renal concerns.

One of the key aspects of the Renal Reset Cookbook is its focus on ingredients that are kidney-friendly. Since individuals with kidney problems often need to restrict their intake of certain minerals, including sodium, potassium, and phosphorus, the cookbook offers a variety of recipes that carefully consider these restrictions while ensuring a flavorful and satisfying dining experience.

Breakfast Recipes

Spinach and Feta Egg Muffins:

Ingredients:
- 6 large eggs
- 1 cup fresh spinach, chopped
- 1/2 cup crumbled feta cheese
- 1/4 cup low-potassium milk
- 1/4 teaspoon black pepper
- 1/4 teaspoon garlic powder
- Cooking spray

Instructions:

1. **Preheat the Oven:**
 - Preheat your oven to 350°F (175°C). Lightly grease a muffin tin with cooking spray.

2. **Prepare Spinach:**
 - Sauté chopped spinach in a pan over medium heat until wilted. Set aside to cool.

3. **Whisk Eggs:**
 - In a bowl, whisk together eggs, low-potassium milk, black pepper, and garlic powder until well combined.

4. **Combine Ingredients:**
 - Add the cooled spinach and crumbled feta to the egg mixture. Gently fold until evenly distributed.

5. **Fill Muffin Cups:**
 - Pour the egg mixture into each muffin cup, filling them about 2/3 full.

6. **Bake**:
 - Bake in the preheated oven for 20-25 minutes or until the egg muffins are set and lightly golden on top.

7. **Cool and Serve:**
 - Allow the egg muffins to cool for a few minutes in the tin before transferring them to a wire rack.

8. **Enjoy**:
 - Serve these renal-friendly egg muffins with a side of sliced tomatoes or whole-grain toast for a wholesome breakfast.

Remember to adapt recipes based on your specific dietary needs and consult with a healthcare professional or dietitian for personalized advice.

1. **Egg White Omelette:**
 - Ingredients: Egg whites, spinach, mushrooms, and a sprinkle of low-sodium cheese.
 - Instructions: Whisk egg whites, pour into a pan, add spinach and mushrooms, cook until set, fold, and sprinkle with cheese.

2. **Quinoa Breakfast Bowl:**
 - Ingredients: Cooked quinoa, diced apples, cinnamon, and a drizzle of honey.
 - Instructions: Mix cooked quinoa with diced apples, sprinkle with cinnamon, and drizzle honey on top.

3. **Banana Nut Smoothie**:
 - Ingredients: Banana, low-potassium nut butter (like almond butter), low-potassium milk (rice milk or almond milk), and ice.
 - Instructions: Blend banana, nut butter, and milk until smooth, add ice, and blend again.

4. **Vegetable Hash:**
 - Ingredients: Sweet potatoes, bell peppers, onions, and lean turkey sausage.

- Instructions: Sauté diced sweet potatoes, bell peppers, onions, and turkey sausage until cooked through.

5. **Yogurt Parfait:**
 - Ingredients: Low-fat yogurt, fresh berries, and a sprinkle of low-phosphorus granola.
 Directions: Arrange yogurt, granola, and berries in a glass or bowl.

Remember to consult with a healthcare professional or a dietitian for personalized advice based on individual dietary needs and restrictions.

Lunch and Dinner Ideas

Resetting your renal health through mindful dietary choices is essential, especially when planning meals like lunch and dinner. Individuals with renal concerns often need to monitor their intake of certain nutrients such as sodium, potassium, and phosphorus. Here's a guide to crafting nutritious and delicious lunch and dinner ideas for a renal reset.

Lunch Ideas:

1. **Grilled Chicken Salad:**
Start with a base of fresh leafy greens, add grilled chicken strips, cherry tomatoes, cucumber, and bell peppers. Dress it with a kidney-friendly vinaigrette made with olive oil, lemon juice, and herbs.

2. **Quinoa and Vegetable Bowl:**
Quinoa is high in both protein and fiber. Mix cooked quinoa with steamed vegetables like zucchini, carrots, and green beans. Season with herbs and a squeeze of lemon for flavor.

3. **Vegetable and Lentil Soup**:

Prepare a hearty soup with low-sodium vegetable broth, lentils, and a variety of kidney-friendly vegetables such as kale, carrots, and celery. Season it with herbs like thyme and rosemary.

4. **Turkey Wrap with Avocado:**

Use a whole-grain wrap to make a turkey and avocado wrap. Add fresh lettuce, tomatoes, and a thin spread of low-sodium mayo for moisture.

5. **Salmon and Asparagus Foil Pack**:

Create a simple foil pack with salmon filets and asparagus. Season with herbs and a touch of lemon. Bake for a quick and nutritious lunch option.

Dinner Ideas:

1. **Baked Cod with Lemon and Herbs:**

Cod is a low-phosphorus fish option. Marinate cod filets with lemon, garlic, and herbs, then bake until flaky. Serve with steamed broccoli and quinoa on the side.

2. **Eggplant and Tomato Stew:**

Sauteed eggplant, tomatoes, onions, and garlic
in olive oil. Add low-sodium vegetable broth
and simmer until vegetables are tender.
Season with kidney-friendly herbs like basil
and oregano.

3. **Chicken and Vegetable Stir-Fry:**

Stir-fry chicken breast strips with
kidney-friendly vegetables like bell peppers,
snap peas, and carrots. Use low-sodium soy
sauce and ginger for flavor.

4. **Mushroom and Spinach Risotto:**

Make a creamy risotto using arborio rice,
mushrooms, and spinach. Use low-sodium
vegetable broth and limit the amount of
Parmesan cheese to control phosphorus
intake.

5. **Grilled Shrimp Skewers:**

Marinate shrimp with olive oil, garlic, and
herbs. Skewer them and grill until cooked.
Serve with a side of steamed asparagus and a
lemon wedge.

General Tips for Renal-Friendly Meals:

Portion Control: Keep portions in check to avoid excess intake of nutrients like potassium and phosphorus.

Limit Processed Foods: Reduce the consumption of processed and packaged foods, as they often contain high levels of sodium and phosphorus additives.

Choose Fresh Ingredients: Opt for fresh fruits and vegetables, lean proteins, and whole grains. Fresh ingredients are lower in sodium and phosphorus compared to processed alternatives.

Stay Hydrated: Adequate hydration is crucial for kidney health. Drink water throughout the day, and consider incorporating hydrating foods like cucumbers and watermelon.

 Consult a Dietitian: Individual dietary needs vary, so it's essential to consult with a renal dietitian. They can provide personalized guidance based on your specific health conditions and requirements.

Crafting renal-friendly lunch and dinner options involves creativity and an understanding of nutrient restrictions. By focusing on fresh, whole foods and mindful seasoning, you can enjoy flavorful meals that support your renal health.

Snacks and Desserts

Maintaining a renal-friendly diet is crucial for individuals with kidney concerns, and careful consideration of snacks and desserts can significantly contribute to a renal reset. The goal is to choose options that are low in potassium, phosphorus, and sodium, key elements that can impact kidney health.

Snack Suggestions:

1. **Fresh Fruits:**
 Embrace fruits with lower potassium content, such as berries (strawberries, blueberries, raspberries) and apples. These can be enjoyed on their own or paired with a dollop of low-phosphorus whipped cream for added flavor.

2. **Vegetable Sticks with Hummus:**
 Snack on crunchy vegetable sticks like carrots, celery, and bell peppers accompanied by a side of homemade hummus. Opt for a hummus recipe that uses low-phosphorus ingredients to keep it kidney-friendly.

3. **Unsalted Nuts**:
 Choose unsalted nuts like almonds, cashews, or walnuts for a satisfying and kidney-friendly

snack. Nuts provide healthy fats and protein without the added sodium, making them a nutritious choice.

4. **Popcorn**:
 Air-popped popcorn is a low-phosphorus and low-sodium snack that can be customized with kidney-friendly seasonings like herbs or a sprinkle of nutritional yeast for added flavor.

5. **Rice Cakes with Cream Cheese:**
 Enjoy rice cakes with a spread of low-fat cream cheese. This combination offers a satisfying crunch and a touch of creaminess without overloading on phosphorus.

Dessert Suggestions:

1. **Gelatin Desserts:**
 Gelatin desserts are a refreshing and kidney-friendly option. Create fruit-infused gelatin with fruits like peaches or pineapple, keeping in mind their lower potassium content.

2. **Sorbet**:
 Indulge in the sweetness of sorbet as a low-potassium alternative to traditional ice cream. Opt for flavors like lemon, lime, or raspberry, and check labels to ensure minimal phosphorus additives.

3. **Rice Pudding with Cinnamon**:
 Prepare a homemade rice pudding using low-phosphorus rice and unsweetened almond milk. Sprinkle it with a dash of cinnamon for added flavor without compromising kidney health.

4. **Angel Food Cake with Berries:**
 Angel food cake is a light and airy dessert that pairs well with fresh berries. Choose berries with lower potassium levels, such as strawberries or blueberries, for a delightful treat.

5. **Peach or Apple Crisp:**
 Bake a kidney-friendly crisp using peaches or apples with a crumbly topping made from oats, flour, and a touch of butter. This provides a comforting dessert with controlled phosphorus content.

6. **Low-Phosphorus Yogurt Parfait:**
 Create a yogurt parfait using low-phosphorus yogurt, granola with limited phosphorus, and sliced bananas or other fruits with moderate potassium levels. This layered dessert offers a variety of textures and flavors.

Remember, individual dietary needs may vary, and it's essential to consult with a healthcare professional or a registered dietitian to tailor these snack and dessert suggestions to your specific renal requirements. They can provide personalized guidance based on your health status and help you make informed choices that support kidney function while still allowing for enjoyable and satisfying snacks and desserts.

CHAPTER 7

Dining Out with Renal Restrictions

Managing rental restrictions while dining out can present challenges, but with careful consideration and awareness, it's possible to enjoy a satisfying and flavorful culinary experience. Individuals with renal issues need to be mindful of their diet to maintain kidney health, and making informed choices when dining out is crucial in this journey. This article explores practical tips and considerations for those navigating the world of dining with renal restrictions.

Understanding Renal Restrictions:

Renal restrictions typically involve limitations on certain nutrients such as sodium, potassium, and phosphorus. These restrictions aim to ease the burden on the kidneys and slow down the progression of kidney disease. When dining out, individuals with renal restrictions must pay attention to menu choices, cooking methods, and ingredient compositions to ensure they align with their dietary needs.

Choosing the Right Restaurant:

Selecting a restaurant that offers a variety of options and is willing to accommodate dietary restrictions is a crucial first step. Many establishments are becoming more aware of the diverse dietary needs of their customers, so don't hesitate to inquire about menu modifications. Opt for restaurants that emphasize fresh, whole ingredients, as these are generally more adaptable to specific dietary requirements.

Menu Exploration:

Once seated, take time to carefully review the menu. Look for dishes that are grilled, baked, or steamed, as these cooking methods typically use less added salt and fat. Avoid fried and heavily processed options, as they often contain higher levels of sodium and phosphorus. Additionally, inquire about the possibility of modifying dishes to meet your specific dietary needs. Many chefs are willing to accommodate requests for adjustments.

Sodium Sensitivity:

Sodium is a major concern for individuals with renal restrictions, as excessive intake can contribute to fluid retention and high blood pressure. When dining out, opt for dishes with minimal added salt. Request that your meal be prepared with little or no added salt, and inquire about low-sodium seasoning alternatives. Be cautious of condiments and sauces, as they can be hidden sources of sodium.

Potassium Management:

For those with renal restrictions, controlling potassium intake is vital. Choose fruits and vegetables that are lower in potassium, such as apples, berries, and green beans. When ordering, request substitutions for high-potassium items and be mindful of portion sizes. Grains, lean proteins, and certain dairy alternatives can be excellent choices for a well-balanced meal without excessive potassium.

Phosphorus Awareness:

Maintaining appropriate phosphorus levels is essential for kidney health. Limiting dairy, processed foods, and certain beverages can help achieve this. When dining out, inquire about phosphorus content in menu items and choose dishes that are naturally lower in phosphorus. Opt for fresh and simple preparations to minimize hidden sources of phosphorus often found in processed foods.

Communication with Staff:

Effective communication with restaurant staff is key to ensuring a positive dining experience. Don't hesitate to inform your server about your dietary restrictions and ask for assistance in making suitable choices. Most establishments are willing to accommodate dietary needs, and clear communication can help avoid misunderstandings.

Beverage Choices:

While water is generally the best choice for hydration, individuals with renal restrictions may need to limit their fluid intake. Opt for water with a slice of lemon or lime for flavor, and be cautious of excessive consumption of caffeinated and sugary beverages. Alcohol should be consumed in moderation, as it can contribute to dehydration and may interact with certain medications.

In conclusion, Dining out with renal restrictions requires careful planning and communication, but it doesn't mean sacrificing flavor and enjoyment. By selecting the right restaurants, exploring menus with awareness, and communicating effectively with staff, individuals with renal restrictions can savor a diverse range of delicious and kidney-friendly meals. Embracing a mindful approach to dining out ensures that the culinary journey remains both pleasurable and health-conscious.

Making Wise Choices at Restaurants

When it comes to making wise choices at a restaurant for renal reset, every decision counts in nurturing your well-being. The journey toward renal health involves a delicate interplay of dietary considerations, and the choices made in a restaurant setting can significantly impact this path. As you navigate through the menu, armed with the knowledge of what's beneficial and what should be approached with caution, you embark on a culinary adventure that not only tantalizes your taste buds but also contributes to the revitalization of your renal function.

Begin this gastronomic expedition by embracing the power of knowledge. Understanding the basics of a renal-friendly diet provides the foundation for making informed choices. Sodium, potassium, phosphorus – these become the watchwords as you scrutinize the menu. Awareness of these dietary components enables you to navigate through the intricate maze of options, steering clear of potential pitfalls that could jeopardize your renal health.

In the realm of sodium, moderation is the key. Restaurants often liberally use salt to enhance flavors, but for renal health, it's imperative to be discerning. Opting for dishes with minimal added salt or requesting the chef to prepare your meal with reduced sodium ensures you savor the essence of the cuisine without compromising your renal objectives.

Turning the spotlight on potassium, it's essential to strike a delicate balance. While potassium is a vital nutrient, excessive intake can pose challenges for those with compromised kidney function. Restaurants frequently feature potassium-rich ingredients, such as tomatoes and potatoes. Opting for alternatives or requesting substitutions showcases your commitment to making choices aligned with your renal goals.

Phosphorus, another player in the intricate dance of renal nutrition, demands attention. Many restaurant offerings boast ingredients rich in phosphorus, such as dairy products and certain proteins. Delving into the menu with a discerning eye allows you to identify and embrace alternatives that promote renal well-being, steering clear of potential phosphorus pitfalls.

As the menu unfolds before you, consider the allure of fresh, vibrant vegetables. Embracing a plant-based focus aligns with the principles of a renal-friendly diet. Crisp salads, steamed vegetables, and other plant-based options not only contribute to your nutritional goals but also infuse your dining experience with a spectrum of colors and textures.

Protein, a cornerstone of any diet, assumes a nuanced role in the context of renal health. Opting for lean protein sources, such as poultry or fish, and avoiding excessively processed or cured meats demonstrate a thoughtful approach to maintaining a delicate equilibrium. Engaging in a dialogue with the restaurant staff, expressing your dietary preferences and restrictions, allows for a customized dining experience that caters to your rental needs.

Navigating the world of beverages becomes a crucial aspect of the restaurant dining experience. Water, an elixir of life, takes center stage. Staying well-hydrated supports kidney function and aids in flushing out toxins. While it's tempting to indulge in sugary or caffeinated beverages, opting for water or herbal teas cultivates a beverage repertoire that nurtures rather than hinders renal health.

Dessert, often the grand finale of a dining experience, beckons with its sweet temptations. However, the savvy diner recognizes the need for moderation in sugar intake. Exploring dessert options that align with your renal goals, such as fruit-based delights or sorbets, allows you to conclude your meal on a sweet note without compromising your dietary objectives.

The ambiance of the restaurant, the interplay of aromas, and the visual feast presented on your plate contribute to the holistic dining experience. Beyond the tangible aspects of the menu, the intangible elements of mindful eating come into play. Taking the time to savor each bite, to relish the textures and flavors, fosters a connection between food and well-being. In this mindful approach, you not only nourish your body but also cultivate a sense of appreciation for the intricate dance of ingredients that contribute to your renal reset.

In the tapestry of restaurant dining, communication emerges as a powerful thread. Engaging with the restaurant staff, communicating your dietary preferences and restrictions, transforms the dining experience into a collaborative endeavor. A chef willing to customize a dish to suit your rental needs becomes a partner in your journey toward optimal health. This collaborative spirit extends beyond the immediate dining encounter, creating an environment where individuals with renal considerations feel supported in their quest for gastronomic satisfaction without compromising well-being.

In conclusion, making wise choices at a restaurant for renal reset transcends the realm of mere culinary decisions. It becomes a conscious, intentional act of self-care. Armed with knowledge, guided by mindfulness, and facilitated by communication, each choice made in a restaurant setting becomes a step toward nurturing renal health. In this gastronomic journey, the symphony of flavors harmonizes with the principles of renal nutrition, creating a narrative where the pleasure of dining converges with the pursuit of well-being.

Navigating Social Gatherings

Navigating social gatherings when you require renal support can present unique challenges, but with careful planning and communication, you can enjoy these events while managing your health needs effectively. Renal support often involves dietary restrictions, fluid intake monitoring, and medication adherence. Here are some practical tips to help you navigate social gatherings while prioritizing your renal health.

1. Communication is Key:
Inform close friends and family about your dietary restrictions and the importance of adhering to your renal support plan. This proactive communication can help create a supportive environment, encouraging others to consider your health needs when planning meals or selecting venues.

2. **Plan Ahead with Hosts:**
If you're attending an event hosted by friends or family, work together to plan a menu that aligns with your renal dietary requirements. Provide them with a list of foods to include or avoid, and share any specific concerns or considerations. Collaboration ensures that

there are suitable options available for you without drawing attention to your health needs during the event.

3. **Bring Your Own Dish:**
Consider preparing a renal-friendly dish to bring to gatherings. This not only guarantees a safe option for you to enjoy but also allows you to contribute to the event, making you an active part of the celebration. Be sure to communicate the ingredients and portion sizes to those who may be interested.

4. **Be Mindful of Fluid Intake:**
Social events often involve beverages, and it's crucial to monitor your fluid intake if you have renal concerns. Opt for small sips, choose beverages wisely, and be aware of hidden liquids in foods like soups and fruits. Communicate your need to manage fluid intake to friends and family so that they can help monitor your consumption during the event.

5. **Choose Wisely from the Menu:**
When attending events at restaurants or other venues, review the menu beforehand if possible. Identify renal-friendly options and inquire about modifications to meet your needs. Don't hesitate to communicate your dietary requirements to the server, ensuring that your meal aligns with your renal support plan.

6. **Educate Others**:
Take the opportunity to educate friends and acquaintances about renal health and the reasons behind your dietary choices. By fostering understanding, you create a supportive social circle that considers your needs when planning gatherings or meals.

7. **Prioritize Medication Adherence:**
If your renal support plan includes medication, ensure that you have a discreet and convenient way to take your medication during social events. Plan ahead by carrying the necessary medications and inform a trusted friend or family member about your schedule, so they can discreetly remind you if needed.

8. **Listen to Your Body:**
Pay attention to how your body responds to different foods and environments. If you experience discomfort or notice changes in your well-being, don't hesitate to take a break or seek a quiet space to address your needs.

In conclusion, navigating social gatherings while managing renal support involves open communication, careful planning, and a proactive approach to your health needs. By working collaboratively with others, educating your social circle, and prioritizing self-care, you can strike a balance between enjoying social events and maintaining your renal health.

CHAPTER 8

Hydration and Kidney Health

Proper hydration is essential for maintaining overall health, and it plays a crucial role in supporting kidney function. The kidneys, two bean-shaped organs located on either side of the spine, are responsible for filtering waste products, excess fluids, and electrolytes from the blood to form urine. Maintaining adequate hydration is vital for these complex physiological processes, as it ensures optimal kidney function and prevents the development of various kidney-related conditions.

The human body is composed of approximately 60% water, emphasizing the fundamental importance of hydration. Water is involved in numerous physiological functions, including nutrient transportation, temperature regulation, and waste elimination. In the context of kidney health, proper hydration helps to dilute urine and prevents the formation of kidney stones, a common condition where solid deposits crystallize in the kidneys.

Dehydration, on the other hand, can have detrimental effects on kidney function. When the body lacks sufficient water, urine becomes concentrated, increasing the risk of kidney stone formation. Additionally, dehydration can lead to a reduction in blood volume, causing the kidneys to work harder to maintain proper fluid balance. Over time, this strain may contribute to the development of chronic kidney disease (CKD), a progressive condition characterized by the gradual loss of kidney function.

One of the key indicators of hydration status is urine color. Clear or light yellow urine generally indicates adequate hydration, while dark yellow or amber-colored urine may suggest dehydration. Monitoring urine color can serve as a simple yet effective method for individuals to assess their hydration levels and make necessary adjustments to their fluid intake.

While water is the primary and most natural source of hydration, other beverages and certain foods also contribute to overall fluid intake. However, it's essential to be mindful of the choices made, as excessive consumption of sugary beverages or those high in caffeine can have adverse effects on kidney health. High sugar intake may contribute to conditions like diabetes, a leading cause of kidney disease, while excessive caffeine consumption can lead to dehydration.

The link between hydration and kidney health becomes even more evident when considering the role of fluid balance in blood pressure regulation. Adequate hydration helps to maintain normal blood volume, supporting optimal blood pressure levels. Hypertension, or high blood pressure, is a significant risk factor for kidney disease. By staying well-hydrated, individuals can contribute to the prevention of hypertension and reduce the strain on their kidneys.

In addition to preventing kidney stones and supporting blood pressure regulation, proper hydration aids in the elimination of waste products from the body. The kidneys filter blood, removing waste and excess fluids to produce urine. Sufficient water intake ensures that this process is efficient, preventing the buildup of toxins in the kidneys and reducing the risk of urinary tract infections.

Certain populations, such as the elderly and individuals with pre-existing health conditions, may be more vulnerable to dehydration and its associated effects on kidney health. Aging can lead to a decreased sense of thirst, making older adults less likely to consume an adequate amount of fluids. Moreover, individuals with conditions like diabetes or heart disease may have specific fluid intake requirements, and careful attention to hydration is crucial for managing their overall health and kidney function.

While hydration is a fundamental aspect of kidney health, it is important to strike a balance. Overhydration, a condition known as hyponatremia, occurs when the balance of electrolytes, particularly sodium, is disrupted by excessive water intake. This condition can lead to symptoms ranging from mild nausea and headache to more severe complications, such as seizures and coma. Therefore, it is essential to consume fluids in moderation and be mindful of individual hydration needs.

In conclusion, maintaining proper hydration is essential for supporting kidney health and preventing a range of kidney-related conditions. Adequate fluid intake helps to prevent the formation of kidney stones, supports blood pressure regulation, and facilitates the efficient elimination of waste products from the body. Monitoring urine color, choosing healthy beverage options, and considering individual hydration needs are all important aspects of promoting optimal kidney function. By recognizing the intricate connection between hydration and kidney health, individuals can take proactive steps to protect and maintain their renal well-being.

Importance of Proper Hydration

Proper hydration plays a pivotal role in maintaining renal health and promoting the efficient functioning of the kidneys. The kidneys are essential organs responsible for filtering waste products and excess fluids from the blood, regulating electrolyte balance, and producing urine. Adequate hydration is crucial for supporting these intricate processes, and it significantly contributes to renal reset – a term used to describe the restoration and optimization of kidney function.

The human body is composed of approximately 60% water, with the kidneys being particularly dependent on proper fluid balance to carry out their functions effectively. Insufficient water intake can lead to dehydration, which may compromise kidney function. When the body is dehydrated, the kidneys receive less blood flow, reducing their ability to filter out waste products. This can result in the accumulation of toxins and metabolic by-products, placing strain on the kidneys and potentially leading to kidney stones or other renal issues.

Hydration is essential for maintaining optimal blood volume and blood pressure, both of which are critical for the kidneys' filtration process. When the body is well-hydrated, blood flows freely through the vessels, enabling the kidneys to efficiently remove waste and excess fluids. Inadequate hydration can lead to a decrease in blood volume, causing the kidneys to conserve water and concentrate urine. This concentrated urine may contribute to the formation of kidney stones, a painful condition arising from the crystallization of minerals in the urine.

Proper hydration also supports the prevention of urinary tract infections (UTIs), a common concern that can affect the kidneys. Drinking an ample amount of water helps flush out bacteria and prevents their colonization in the urinary tract. This is particularly crucial for renal health, as untreated UTIs can progress to kidney infections, posing a more severe threat to renal function.

Moreover, sufficient water intake plays a role in preventing the development of chronic kidney disease (CKD). Chronic dehydration over time can lead to sustained stress on the kidneys, potentially contributing to the progression of renal dysfunction. Individuals with pre-existing kidney conditions, such as polycystic kidney disease or diabetes, are especially vulnerable, and maintaining proper hydration becomes even more crucial in managing and mitigating the impact of these conditions on renal health.

Renal reset, in the context of hydration, refers to the ability of the kidneys to restore and optimize their function when provided with adequate fluids. Hydration acts as a reset button for the renal system, allowing the kidneys to efficiently filter blood, balance electrolytes, and eliminate waste products. Regular and adequate water intake supports the kidneys in maintaining their delicate equilibrium, preventing the buildup of harmful substances that could compromise their function.

In conclusion, the importance of proper hydration for renal reset cannot be overstated. Water is the foundation of kidney health, and maintaining an appropriate fluid balance is essential for the kidneys to function optimally. Adequate hydration supports the prevention of kidney stones, urinary tract infections, and chronic kidney disease. By understanding and prioritizing the role of hydration in renal health, individuals can take proactive steps to ensure the well-being of their kidneys and promote overall physiological balance.

Choosing the Right Beverages

Choosing the right beverages for renal support is crucial for individuals with kidney issues, as it plays a significant role in managing kidney function and overall health. The kidneys are essential organs responsible for filtering waste products and excess fluids from the blood, so making wise beverage choices can positively impact kidney function. Here's a comprehensive guide on selecting the right beverages for renal support.

Water is the cornerstone of kidney-friendly beverages. Staying well-hydrated is essential for maintaining kidney health, as it helps in flushing out toxins and preventing the formation of kidney stones. Adequate water intake can also prevent dehydration, which can strain the kidneys. However, the amount of water needed varies among individuals, so consulting a healthcare professional for personalized advice is recommended.

Herbal teas are excellent alternatives to caffeinated beverages. Many herbal teas, such as dandelion and nettle tea, are known for their diuretic properties, promoting fluid balance without the added stress of caffeine. These teas are not only hydrating but also provide

additional health benefits, like
anti-inflammatory and antioxidant properties.

Fruit juices can be a part of a renal-friendly
beverage plan, but it's crucial to choose
carefully. Opt for juices that are lower in
potassium and phosphorus, as high levels of
these minerals can be harmful to individuals
with kidney issues. Apple and cranberry juices
are generally good choices, as they are lower
in potassium and phosphorus compared to
citrus juices.

Vegetable juices, particularly those made from
kidney-friendly vegetables like cucumber and
celery, can also be incorporated into a renal
support beverage plan. These juices provide
essential vitamins and minerals without
overloading the kidneys with excessive
amounts of potassium and phosphorus.

Milk and dairy products are common sources
of protein and calcium, but individuals with
kidney issues need to be mindful of their
intake. Choose low-fat or fat-free dairy options
to reduce saturated fat content. Additionally,
considering dairy alternatives like almond or
rice milk can be a suitable option for those with
lactose intolerance or a need for lower
phosphorus levels.

Sports drinks and sodas should be limited or avoided, as they often contain high levels of phosphorus and added sugars. These beverages can contribute to dehydration and may exacerbate kidney issues. Opting for water or herbal teas is a much healthier choice for individuals with compromised kidney function.

Alcohol consumption should be moderated, as excessive alcohol intake can lead to dehydration and negatively impact kidney function. If consumed, it's essential to do so in moderation and be mindful of the potential interaction with medications that individuals with kidney issues may be taking.

Limiting caffeine intake is advisable for those with kidney concerns. While moderate caffeine consumption is generally considered safe, excessive caffeine can lead to dehydration and may elevate blood pressure, putting additional stress on the kidneys. Choosing decaffeinated coffee or herbal teas can be a better option for renal support.

Sugar-free beverages may seem like a suitable choice for individuals with kidney issues, but it's essential to be cautious. Some sugar substitutes may contain phosphorus, which can be problematic for those with compromised kidney function. Reading labels and choosing beverages with phosphorus-free sweeteners is crucial.

In summary, choosing the right beverages for renal support involves making mindful and informed choices to promote kidney health. Water, herbal teas, and carefully selected fruit and vegetable juices can contribute to hydration and provide additional health benefits. It's essential to avoid or limit the consumption of beverages high in phosphorus, potassium, and added sugars, such as sodas and certain fruit juices. Consulting with a healthcare professional or a registered dietitian can provide personalized guidance to create a beverage plan that supports kidney function and overall well-being.

CHAPTER 9

Managing Special Dietary Needs

Managing special dietary needs for renal reset involves careful consideration of nutrition to support kidney health. Renal reset refers to the process of resetting and optimizing kidney function through lifestyle changes, with a primary focus on diet. Individuals with renal issues, such as chronic kidney disease (CKD), require specific dietary adjustments to manage their condition effectively.

The foundation of a renal-friendly diet revolves around controlling key nutrients like sodium, potassium, phosphorus, and protein. Sodium restriction is crucial to manage blood pressure, a common concern for those with kidney problems. This involves limiting the intake of processed foods and avoiding high-sodium seasonings. Instead, opting for fresh herbs and spices can add flavor without compromising kidney health.

Potassium is another essential nutrient that requires careful monitoring. While potassium is vital for nerve and muscle function, excess levels can be harmful to individuals with compromised kidney function. High-potassium foods, such as bananas and oranges, may need moderation or substitution with lower-potassium alternatives.

Phosphorus management is vital as well. Elevated phosphorus levels can lead to bone and cardiovascular issues in individuals with kidney disease. Foods rich in phosphorus, like dairy products and certain meats, should be limited. Reading food labels becomes crucial for identifying hidden phosphorus in processed items.

Protein intake is a key aspect of renal nutrition. While protein is essential for overall health, excessive protein can strain the kidneys. In renal reset, the focus is on maintaining an adequate but not excessive protein intake. High-quality protein sources like lean meats, fish, and eggs are preferred over processed or red meats. Plant-based protein options such as legumes and tofu can also be incorporated.

Adequate fluid intake is fundamental for kidney health. Staying hydrated helps the kidneys flush out waste products efficiently. However, fluid restriction may be necessary for some individuals with advanced kidney disease, depending on their specific condition. Balancing fluid intake with individual needs is crucial in managing renal reset.

In addition to monitoring specific nutrients, portion control plays a significant role in renal reset. Controlling portion sizes helps manage overall nutrient intake and prevents overloading the kidneys. Working with a healthcare professional or a registered dietitian is advisable to create personalized meal plans that align with individual health needs and preferences.

Beyond nutrient management, adopting a heart-healthy diet is beneficial for individuals with renal concerns. This involves incorporating fruits, vegetables, whole grains, and healthy fats while limiting saturated and trans fats. Maintaining a healthy weight and engaging in regular physical activity contribute to overall well-being and can positively impact kidney health.

Educating individuals undergoing renal reset and their families is essential for long-term success. Understanding the rationale behind dietary recommendations empowers individuals to make informed choices. Regular follow-ups with healthcare providers allow for adjustments to the dietary plan based on individual progress and changing health needs.

Social support is a crucial component of managing special dietary needs for renal reset. Family and friends play a vital role in creating a supportive environment, ensuring adherence to dietary restrictions, and promoting overall well-being. Encouraging open communication and addressing any challenges or concerns can enhance the success of renal reset.

In conclusion, managing special dietary needs for renal reset involves a comprehensive approach that considers various aspects of nutrition, lifestyle, and individual preferences. By focusing on controlling sodium, potassium, phosphorus, and protein intake, along with maintaining fluid balance and adopting a heart-healthy diet, individuals with renal concerns can work towards optimizing kidney function. Collaboration with healthcare professionals, ongoing education, and strong social support are integral components of successful renal reset, empowering individuals to take control of their health and well-being.

Renal Diets for Specific Conditions

Renal diets play a crucial role in managing various kidney-related conditions. These specialized diets are designed to alleviate symptoms, slow disease progression, and improve overall kidney function. Tailoring dietary choices to specific conditions is essential, as different kidney issues require varying nutritional approaches.

Chronic Kidney Disease (CKD):
Individuals with CKD often need to monitor their protein, phosphorus, potassium, and sodium intake. Reducing protein helps minimize the strain on the kidneys, while controlling phosphorus is vital to prevent bone and cardiovascular complications. Potassium levels must be regulated to prevent electrolyte imbalances, and sodium intake is often restricted to manage blood pressure.

A CKD-friendly diet typically includes lean protein sources like poultry and fish, limited dairy, and phosphorus-conscious choices such as low-phosphorus grains. Controlling fluid intake is also crucial for managing fluid retention, a common issue in CKD.

Diabetic Nephropathy:
For those with diabetic nephropathy, managing blood sugar levels is paramount. A diet focusing on complex carbohydrates, high-fiber foods, and moderate protein helps control glucose levels. Limiting added sugars and refined carbohydrates aids in preventing blood sugar spikes, subsequently reducing the risk of kidney damage.

Additionally, monitoring blood pressure is crucial for individuals with diabetic nephropathy. A diet low in sodium and rich in potassium, through fruits and vegetables, contributes to blood pressure management.

Hypertensive Nephropathy:
Hypertensive nephropathy, often caused by prolonged high blood pressure, requires a diet aimed at reducing hypertension. Sodium restriction is vital, as excess sodium can elevate blood pressure. Potassium-rich foods, such as bananas and sweet potatoes, play a role in counteracting the effects of sodium.

Healthy fats, found in avocados and olive oil, contribute to cardiovascular health. Maintaining a healthy weight through portion control and regular exercise is also emphasized to manage blood pressure effectively.

Polycystic Kidney Disease (PKD):

PKD is a genetic disorder characterized by fluid-filled cysts in the kidneys. While there isn't a specific diet to cure PKD, certain dietary modifications can help manage symptoms. Maintaining hydration is crucial to prevent kidney stones, a common complication.

A low-sodium diet helps control blood pressure, reducing the strain on cyst-filled kidneys. Adequate protein intake, with a focus on high-quality sources, supports overall health. Regular monitoring of phosphorus and potassium levels is advised, as imbalances can occur.

Nephrotic Syndrome:
Individuals with nephrotic syndrome often experience protein leakage in the urine, leading to low protein levels in the blood. A diet with increased protein intake may be recommended to address this deficiency. However, the source of protein is crucial, favoring high-quality options like eggs, fish, and lean meats.

Sodium restriction is essential to manage edema, a common symptom of nephrotic syndrome. Diuretic foods, such as celery and watermelon, can complement medication in controlling fluid retention.

In conclusion, renal diets for specific conditions are tailored to address the unique needs of individuals with kidney-related issues. These diets prioritize the control of protein, phosphorus, potassium, sodium, and other nutrients based on the underlying condition. While there are commonalities, such as the emphasis on whole, nutrient-dense foods, the nuances in each diet highlight the importance of personalized nutrition in managing renal health. It is crucial for individuals to work closely with healthcare professionals and registered dietitians to create a comprehensive and effective dietary plan that suits their specific condition and health goals.

Tips for Vegetarian and Vegan Options

Choosing vegetarian and vegan options while managing renal health requires careful consideration to ensure a balanced and nutrient-rich diet. Individuals with renal issues need to monitor their protein, phosphorus, potassium, and sodium intake. Here are some tips for incorporating vegetarian and vegan choices into a renal-friendly diet:

1. Protein Sources:
- Opt for plant-based protein sources like legumes (lentils, chickpeas, and black beans), tofu, tempeh, and edamame.
- Include whole grains such as quinoa, bulgur, and farro to boost protein intake.
- Experiment with meat substitutes made from soy or pea protein but check labels for phosphorus content.

2. Portion Control:
- Be mindful of portion sizes to avoid excessive protein intake, which can strain the kidneys.
- Consider consulting a dietitian to determine the appropriate amount of protein for your specific needs.

3. Limit Phosphorus-Rich Foods:
- Many plant-based foods contain phosphorus, so it's essential to be aware of phosphorus content.
- Choose lower phosphorus plant-based options like white bread over whole grain and rice over bran.

4. Watch Potassium Intake:
- Some plant-based foods are high in potassium, including bananas, oranges, and tomatoes.
- Moderation is key; consider smaller servings or choose lower-potassium alternatives.

5. Calcium Considerations:
- Dairy is a common source of calcium, but there are plant-based options like fortified plant milk, tofu, and leafy greens.
- Ensure an adequate calcium intake while managing phosphorus levels.

6. Fluid Management:
- Stay hydrated, but be mindful of fluid intake based on individual needs and medical advice.
- Limit beverages high in phosphorus and potassium, such as certain fruit juices.

7. Mindful Cooking Methods:
- Opt for cooking methods that preserve nutrients without adding unnecessary

elements. Steaming, baking, and grilling are good choices.
 - Avoid excessive salt when seasoning; consider using herbs and spices for flavor.

8. **Label Reading:
 - Check food labels for phosphorus and potassium content, as manufacturers may add these minerals during processing.
 - Familiarize yourself with the various names for additives that contribute to phosphorus levels.

9. Diversify Your Diet:
 - Incorporate a variety of fruits, vegetables, and grains to ensure a broad spectrum of nutrients.
 - Rotate your food choices to prevent monotony and ensure a well-rounded intake.

10. Supplementation Guidance:
 - Consult with a healthcare professional or dietitian to determine if supplementation is necessary, especially for nutrients like B12, iron, and omega-3 fatty acids.

11. Meal Planning:
 - Plan meals in advance to ensure a balanced distribution of nutrients throughout the day.
 - This can help prevent overconsumption of specific minerals during a single meal.

12. Consult a Dietitian:
 - Every individual's nutritional needs are unique, especially when managing renal health. A dietitian can provide personalized guidance and ensure nutritional requirements are met.

13. Be Mindful of Hidden Ingredients:
 - Some vegetarian and vegan products may contain high levels of sodium or phosphorus as additives. Check ingredient lists thoroughly.

14. Maintain a Food Diary:
 - Keep a record of your meals, snacks, and fluid intake to identify patterns and make adjustments if needed.

15. Educate Yourself:
 - Stay informed about renal-friendly vegetarian and vegan options. Attend workshops, read reputable sources, and engage with healthcare professionals for ongoing education.

In conclusion, adopting a vegetarian or vegan diet while managing renal health is feasible with careful planning and attention to nutrient intake. Consulting healthcare professionals, especially dietitians, is crucial for personalized guidance. By incorporating a diverse range of plant-based foods and being mindful of specific nutrient levels, individuals can enjoy a satisfying and nourishing diet that supports renal health.

CHAPTER 10

Exercise and Kidney Wellness

Regular exercise plays a crucial role in maintaining overall health, and its positive impact extends to kidney wellness as well. The kidneys, vital organs in the human body, are responsible for filtering waste products and excess fluids from the blood, regulating blood pressure, and maintaining electrolyte balance. Engaging in physical activity has been shown to contribute significantly to kidney health by promoting proper blood flow, reducing the risk of chronic kidney disease (CKD), and supporting overall well-being.

One of the primary benefits of exercise for kidney wellness is its role in managing and preventing various risk factors associated with kidney problems. Conditions such as hypertension and diabetes are leading causes of CKD, and exercise has been proven effective in controlling both. Regular physical activity helps regulate blood pressure by improving the elasticity of blood vessels and reducing the workload on the heart. Moreover, exercise enhances insulin sensitivity, which is crucial in preventing and managing diabetes, a major contributor to kidney disease.

Maintaining a healthy weight is another key aspect of kidney wellness, and exercise is a cornerstone in achieving and sustaining this goal. Obesity is a known risk factor for kidney disease, as it is associated with the development of conditions like diabetes and hypertension. Regular physical activity helps in weight management by burning calories, building muscle mass, and boosting metabolism. This, in turn, reduces the risk of obesity-related complications that could negatively impact kidney function.

Beyond weight management, exercise contributes to the overall cardiovascular health that is closely linked to kidney function. Cardiovascular exercises, such as running, swimming, and cycling, improve the efficiency of the heart and lungs, ensuring an adequate supply of oxygen-rich blood to all organs, including the kidneys. Adequate blood flow is essential for the filtration process in the kidneys, and regular exercise helps maintain optimal cardiovascular function.

In addition to its role in preventing kidney disease, exercise has shown promise in managing existing kidney conditions. Individuals with CKD often experience fatigue and reduced physical function, making it challenging to engage in regular activities. However, tailored exercise programs have been designed to address the specific needs and limitations of individuals with kidney disease. These programs aim to improve muscle strength, endurance, and overall physical well-being, ultimately enhancing the quality of life for those with compromised kidney function.

It's important to note that the type and intensity of exercise should be adapted to individual health conditions. Consultation with healthcare professionals, particularly for individuals with existing kidney disease, is crucial to ensure that the exercise regimen is safe and beneficial. In some cases, modifications to the intensity or type of exercise may be necessary to accommodate the specific needs and limitations of individuals with kidney issues.

Hydration is another crucial aspect of kidney health, and exercise can impact fluid balance in the body. While staying hydrated is important, excessive fluid loss through sweating during intense physical activity may pose risks for individuals with kidney problems. Therefore, it is essential to strike a balance and adjust fluid intake accordingly, especially for those with kidney conditions.

In summary, exercise plays a multifaceted role in promoting kidney wellness. It addresses key risk factors such as hypertension and diabetes, supports weight management, enhances cardiovascular health, and contributes to overall well-being. Tailored exercise programs can also benefit individuals with existing kidney conditions by improving their physical function and quality of life. However, it's essential to approach exercise with awareness of individual health status, seeking guidance from healthcare professionals to ensure a safe and effective fitness routine that aligns with kidney health goals.

Incorporating Physical Activity

Incorporating physical activity into one's lifestyle plays a pivotal role in promoting overall health, and this principle extends to renal health as well. The kidneys, essential organs for filtering waste and excess fluids from the blood, benefit significantly from regular physical activity. Engaging in appropriate exercises can contribute to maintaining kidney function, preventing certain renal conditions, and improving overall well-being.

Chronic Kidney Disease (CKD) is a prevalent health issue globally, affecting millions of people. Physical activity has emerged as a non-pharmacological intervention that can mitigate the risk factors associated with CKD. Regular exercise helps manage conditions such as hypertension and diabetes, both of which are primary contributors to kidney dysfunction. By promoting cardiovascular health and controlling blood sugar levels, physical activity indirectly safeguards the kidneys from potential damage.

Moreover, exercise contributes to weight management, another crucial factor in renal health. Obesity is a known risk factor for kidney disease, and maintaining a healthy weight through regular physical activity helps reduce this risk. Additionally, exercise aids in the prevention of metabolic syndrome, a cluster of conditions that includes abdominal obesity, high blood pressure, and insulin resistance, all of which elevate the risk of developing kidney disease.

The benefits of physical activity on renal health extend beyond prevention, encompassing the management of existing kidney conditions. Individuals with CKD often face complications like muscle wasting and reduced physical function. Incorporating appropriate exercises tailored to the individual's health status can mitigate these complications, enhancing muscular strength and overall functional capacity.

Aerobic exercises, such as walking, cycling, or swimming, are particularly beneficial for individuals with kidney disease. These activities improve cardiovascular fitness, leading to better blood circulation and oxygenation of tissues, including the kidneys. Resistance training, involving activities like weight lifting, contributes to muscle strength, which is crucial for those with compromised physical function due to kidney-related issues.

However, it is essential for individuals with kidney disease to consult with healthcare professionals before embarking on a new exercise regimen. Certain exercises may need to be modified based on the individual's health status, and close monitoring is crucial to prevent potential complications. Additionally, hydration plays a vital role in kidney health, and individuals engaging in physical activity must ensure adequate fluid intake, especially if there are any restrictions on water consumption due to kidney conditions.

In the realm of renal health, physical activity extends its positive influence even to those undergoing dialysis. While dialysis is a life-saving intervention for individuals with advanced kidney disease, it can lead to physical deconditioning. Incorporating light to moderate-intensity exercises into the routine of dialysis patients has been shown to improve physical function, reduce fatigue, and enhance overall quality of life.

Furthermore, the psychological benefits of regular physical activity should not be overlooked in the context of renal health. Dealing with chronic conditions such as CKD can be mentally challenging, and exercise has been proven to have positive effects on mood and mental well-being. The release of endorphins during physical activity can alleviate symptoms of anxiety and depression, fostering a more positive outlook on managing chronic kidney conditions.

In conclusion, incorporating physical activity into one's lifestyle is a valuable and multifaceted approach to promoting renal health. Whether in preventing the onset of kidney disease or managing existing conditions, exercise proves to be a powerful tool. Tailoring exercise regimens to individual health status, consulting healthcare professionals, and ensuring proper hydration are crucial elements in realizing the full benefits of physical activity on renal health. As we strive for holistic well-being, recognizing the interplay between regular exercise and kidney health is a significant step towards fostering a healthier, more active future.

Tips for Vegetarian and Vegan Options

A renal diet is crucial for individuals with kidney issues, as it helps manage the intake of certain nutrients to maintain kidney function. For vegetarians and vegans, navigating a renal diet can be challenging due to restrictions on various foods. However, with thoughtful planning and attention to nutrient intake, it is possible to adhere to a renal diet while following a plant-based lifestyle. Here are some tips for incorporating vegetarian and vegan options into a renal diet:

Understanding the Renal Diet for Vegetarians and Vegans

1. **Monitor Protein Intake:**
 - Opt for plant-based protein sources such as legumes, beans, lentils, and tofu.
 - Pay attention to the quantity of protein consumed, as excessive protein can strain the kidneys.

2. **Quality of Protein Matters:**
 - Choose high-quality plant proteins to ensure a balanced amino acid profile.
 - Quinoa, chia seeds, and hemp seeds are excellent sources of complete proteins.

3. Control Phosphorus Intake:
 - Many plant-based foods contain phosphorus, but in a less absorbable form. Still, monitoring intake is important.
 - Limit high-phosphorus foods like nuts, seeds, and whole grains.

4. Calcium Sources:
 - Incorporate calcium-rich plant foods like kale, collard greens, broccoli, and fortified plant-based milk alternatives.

5. Potassium Management:
 - Potassium is abundant in vegetables and fruits.Choose low-potassium options, such as berries, apples, and cauliflower.
 - Cooking methods like leaching can help reduce potassium content in certain vegetables.

6. Fluid Intake:
 - Adequate hydration is crucial. Monitor fluid intake and choose hydrating foods like water-rich fruits and vegetables.

7. Limit Sodium:
 - Processed and canned vegetarian or vegan products may be high in sodium. Opt for fresh, whole foods and use herbs and spices for flavor.

Meal Planning for Renal-Friendly Vegetarian and Vegan Diets

8. Portion Control:
 - Be mindful of portion sizes to manage nutrient intake effectively.

9. Balanced Meals:
 - Create balanced meals with a combination of carbohydrates, proteins, and healthy fats.
 - Consider consulting a dietitian to ensure all essential nutrients are included.

10. Snacking Smartly:
 - Choose renal-friendly snacks like fresh fruits, air-popped popcorn, or vegetable sticks with hummus.

11. Reading Labels:
 - Scrutinize food labels for phosphorus and sodium content.
 - Be aware of hidden sources of these minerals in processed vegetarian and vegan products.

12. Experiment with Grains:
 - Explore grains like bulgur, farro, and couscous as alternatives to high-phosphorus whole grains.

Cooking Techniques for Renal-Friendly Vegetarian and Vegan Dishes

13. Leaching Phosphorus:
 - Leach high-phosphorus foods like beans by soaking them overnight and discarding the soaking water.

14. Use Herbs and Spices:
 - Enhance flavor without added sodium by using herbs, spices, and citrus juices.

15. Grilling and Roasting:
 - Opt for grilling or roasting to enhance flavors without excessive use of oils or salt.

16. Limit Processed Foods:
 - Minimize the consumption of processed vegetarian or vegan products, as they may contain hidden additives.

Consulting Professionals

17. Dietitian Guidance:
 - Seek guidance from a registered dietitian who specializes in vegetarian or vegan diets for kidney health.

18. Regular Monitoring:
 - Regularly monitor blood levels of key nutrients to ensure proper management of the renal diet.

Maintaining a vegetarian or vegan lifestyle while adhering to a renal diet requires careful planning and attention to nutrient intake. By incorporating a variety of plant-based foods, monitoring protein, phosphorus, and potassium levels, and utilizing appropriate cooking techniques, individuals with kidney issues can successfully follow a renal-friendly diet. Consulting with healthcare professionals, especially a dietitian, is essential for personalized guidance and ensuring optimal kidney health while enjoying a plant-based diet.

CHAPTER 11

Exercise and Kidney Wellness

Regular exercise plays a crucial role in maintaining overall health, and its impact extends to the well-being of vital organs, including the kidneys. The kidneys, responsible for filtering waste and excess fluids from the blood, benefit significantly from a physically active lifestyle. This article delves into the intricate relationship between exercise and kidney wellness, exploring how various forms of physical activity contribute to kidney health.

1. Improved Blood Circulation:
One of the primary advantages of regular exercise is the enhancement of blood circulation throughout the body. As the heart pumps blood more efficiently during physical activity, the kidneys receive a steady supply of oxygen and nutrients. This improved circulation aids in the optimal functioning of the kidneys, supporting their essential role in filtering and purifying the blood.

2. Blood Pressure Management:
Exercise is a cornerstone in managing blood pressure, a critical factor in kidney health. Hypertension, or high blood pressure, can

strain the blood vessels in the kidneys, leading to potential damage over time. Engaging in aerobic exercises, such as brisk walking, jogging, or swimming, helps regulate blood pressure and reduces the risk of kidney-related complications.

3. Weight Management:
Maintaining a healthy weight is paramount for kidney wellness. Obesity is linked to an increased risk of kidney disease. Regular exercise, combined with a balanced diet, contributes to weight management and helps prevent the development of conditions like diabetes and metabolic syndrome, which can adversely affect kidney function.

4. Diabetes Prevention and Control:
Type 2 diabetes is a significant risk factor for kidney disease. Exercise plays a pivotal role in preventing and managing diabetes by improving insulin sensitivity and glucose regulation. Activities like strength training and aerobic exercises assist in controlling blood sugar levels, thereby reducing the burden on the kidneys.

5. Enhanced Immune Function:
Exercise has been shown to boost the immune system, which indirectly benefits kidney health. A robust immune system helps the body fend off infections and inflammation, reducing the

likelihood of kidney-related complications. Moderate, consistent exercise has immunomodulatory effects that contribute to overall well-being.

6. Oxidative Stress Reduction:
The kidneys are susceptible to oxidative stress, a condition where the balance between free radicals and antioxidants is disrupted. Regular exercise helps mitigate oxidative stress by promoting the production of antioxidants in the body. This protective mechanism contributes to the preservation of kidney function and reduces the risk of oxidative damage.

7. Fluid Balance and Electrolyte Regulation:
Maintaining the right balance of fluids and electrolytes is crucial for kidney function. Sweating during exercise helps regulate body temperature and facilitates the elimination of excess fluids and salts. Adequate hydration before, during, and after exercise supports the kidneys in maintaining their delicate balance of electrolytes and fluids.

8. Stress Reduction:
Chronic stress can have detrimental effects on overall health, including kidney function. Exercise is a natural stress reliever, triggering the release of endorphins and promoting a sense of well-being. By reducing stress, exercise indirectly supports kidney health and

contributes to a more balanced and resilient physiological state.

9. Renal Blood Flow Enhancement:

Engaging in regular physical activity has been associated with improved renal blood flow. This increased blood flow ensures that the kidneys receive a sufficient oxygen supply, promoting their efficient filtration processes. Activities that elevate heart rate and engage large muscle groups contribute to enhanced renal perfusion.

10. Mitigation of Inflammatory Responses:

Inflammation is a common factor in the progression of kidney diseases. Exercise has anti-inflammatory effects on the body, helping to mitigate chronic inflammation. By reducing inflammation, exercise plays a protective role in preventing conditions that could compromise kidney function over time.

In summary, exercise is a cornerstone of kidney wellness, offering a myriad of benefits that extend beyond physical fitness. From improved blood circulation and blood pressure management to weight control, diabetes prevention, and stress reduction, regular physical activity fosters an environment conducive to optimal kidney function. Incorporating a variety of exercises, including aerobic activities, strength training, and flexibility exercises, can contribute to a holistic approach to kidney health. As with any lifestyle change, it's advisable to consult with healthcare professionals to tailor an exercise regimen that aligns with individual health needs and considerations. Prioritizing regular physical activity is an investment in not only cardiovascular fitness but also the long-term health and well-being of the kidneys.

Incorporating physical activity

Incorporating physical activity into a renal reset regimen is a crucial component for maintaining overall health and well-being, especially for individuals with renal concerns. Renal reset, often associated with the optimization of kidney function, involves lifestyle modifications that extend beyond dietary changes. The inclusion of regular physical activity not only complements these adjustments but also offers a myriad of benefits for renal health.

Exercise has been widely recognized as a cornerstone of a healthy lifestyle, and its impact on renal function is no exception. Engaging in regular physical activity promotes cardiovascular health, helps manage weight, and contributes to improved blood circulation, all of which play a significant role in supporting renal function. For individuals with kidney-related issues, tailoring exercise routines to their specific needs becomes imperative.

One of the key considerations when incorporating physical activity into a renal reset plan is the type and intensity of exercise. Low-impact activities such as walking, cycling, and swimming are often recommended, as they reduce the risk of injury and minimize stress on the kidneys. Strength training, when done with proper guidance and moderation, can also be beneficial in improving muscle mass and overall metabolic health.

Aerobic exercises, known for their cardiovascular benefits, contribute to better blood flow and oxygenation, positively impacting renal function. These exercises can include brisk walking, jogging, or aerobic dance routines. However, it's crucial for individuals to consult their healthcare professionals before starting any exercise program, as the appropriateness of activities may vary based on individual health conditions.

Beyond the physiological benefits, regular physical activity plays a pivotal role in managing risk factors associated with kidney diseases. Hypertension and diabetes, two common risk factors for kidney problems, can be effectively managed through exercise. By promoting weight loss and enhancing insulin sensitivity, physical activity addresses these risk factors, thereby reducing the burden on the kidneys.

In addition to its direct impact on renal health, exercise contributes to an improved quality of life for individuals undergoing a renal reset. The psychological benefits of regular physical activity, including stress reduction and improved mood, are particularly relevant in managing the emotional challenges that often accompany health conditions. Incorporating activities that individuals enjoy ensures a more sustainable and enjoyable exercise routine.

It's important to note that the intensity and duration of exercise should be tailored to an individual's fitness level and health status. Gradual progression, especially for those who have been sedentary or have pre-existing health conditions, is essential to avoid potential complications. Regular monitoring by healthcare professionals is crucial to assess the impact of exercise on renal function and make necessary adjustments to the exercise plan.

Hydration is another critical aspect to consider when integrating physical activity into a renal reset regimen. Staying well-hydrated is essential for individuals with kidney concerns, as it helps flush out waste products and toxins from the body. Proper fluid intake before, during, and after exercise is vital to maintain optimal hydration levels and support kidney function.

In summary, incorporating physical activity into a renal reset plan is a multifaceted approach that requires careful consideration of individual health status and preferences.

From low-impact aerobic exercises to strength training, a well-rounded exercise routine can contribute significantly to overall renal health. Coupled with proper hydration and regular monitoring by healthcare professionals, physical activity becomes a powerful ally in the journey towards renal optimization and improved well-being.

Tailored Exercises for Renal Health

Tailored exercises play a crucial role in promoting renal health, providing individuals with kidney-related concerns a means to enhance their well-being through targeted physical activity. Chronic Kidney Disease (CKD) affects millions globally, necessitating a comprehensive approach to its management. Incorporating tailored exercises into a renal health regimen can yield significant benefits, ranging from improved cardiovascular function to enhanced overall quality of life.

Individuals with CKD often face physical limitations, making it imperative to tailor exercise routines to their specific needs. Low-impact activities such as walking, swimming, and cycling are commonly recommended, as they minimize strain on the kidneys while promoting cardiovascular health. These exercises contribute to maintaining a healthy weight, a critical factor in managing CKD, as obesity is a known risk factor for the progression of kidney disease.

Resistance training also holds promise in renal health. Tailored strength-building exercises help combat muscle wasting, a common complication in CKD. By enhancing muscle mass, individuals can mitigate the physical decline associated with kidney dysfunction. Resistance exercises can be adapted to various fitness levels, allowing for a personalized approach that considers the individual's specific condition and capabilities.

Furthermore, flexibility exercises, such as stretching and yoga, can be beneficial for individuals with renal issues. These activities improve joint mobility and reduce the risk of injuries, addressing some of the challenges CKD patients may face due to decreased physical function. Additionally, incorporating mindfulness through yoga may contribute to managing stress, a factor known to impact kidney health adversely.

Tailoring exercises for renal health also involves considering the individual's stage of CKD. In the early stages, individuals may have fewer physical limitations and can engage in a broader range of activities. As the disease progresses, adjustments become necessary to accommodate changes in stamina, strength, and overall health. Regular monitoring and communication with healthcare professionals are crucial to adapt exercise routines effectively as the condition evolves.

It's important to note that dehydration is a common concern for individuals with kidney issues. Therefore, proper hydration must be emphasized during exercise. Tailored exercise plans should include guidance on fluid intake to ensure that individuals maintain a healthy balance without putting excess strain on their kidneys.

Engaging in tailored exercises for renal health extends beyond the physical realm. Social and emotional well-being is integral to an individual's overall health, especially for those dealing with chronic conditions. Group exercise classes or support groups tailored for individuals with kidney issues can provide a sense of community, motivation, and shared experiences. This social aspect can enhance adherence to exercise routines and contribute to a positive mental outlook.

Moreover, education plays a crucial role in the success of tailored exercise programs for renal health. Individuals should be informed about the specific benefits of exercise for kidney health, as well as the precautions and modifications needed based on their condition. Empowering individuals with knowledge fosters a sense of ownership over their health, promoting a proactive approach to managing CKD through regular physical activity.

In conclusion, tailored exercises are a cornerstone in promoting renal health for individuals with CKD. A personalized approach, considering the individual's physical condition, stage of kidney disease, and overall well-being, can yield significant benefits. From low-impact cardiovascular activities to resistance training and flexibility exercises, a comprehensive exercise plan can contribute to maintaining muscle mass, managing weight, and enhancing overall quality of life. Combining physical activity with proper hydration, social support, and education creates a holistic approach to renal health that empowers individuals in their journey towards well-being despite the challenges of chronic kidney disease.

CHAPTER 12

Regular Health Check-ups

Regular health check-ups are crucial for maintaining renal health and preventing potential complications. The kidneys play a vital role in filtering waste products and excess fluids from the blood, regulating blood pressure, and balancing electrolytes. A routine health check-up specifically focused on renal function can help detect issues early on, allowing for timely intervention and prevention of more severe conditions.

One of the primary components of a renal health check-up is a comprehensive blood test. This test assesses various parameters, including creatinine and blood urea nitrogen (BUN) levels. Elevated amounts of these chemicals may suggest a malfunctioning kidney. Creatinine is a waste product generated by muscle metabolism, and BUN is a byproduct of protein breakdown. When the kidneys are not functioning optimally, these waste products can accumulate in the blood, signaling potential renal dysfunction.

In addition to blood tests, a urine analysis is often included in renal health check-ups. This test evaluates the presence of abnormalities such as proteinuria, hematuria, or the presence of casts. Proteinuria, or the presence of excess protein in the urine, can be a sign of kidney damage. Hematuria, the presence of blood in the urine, may indicate various renal conditions, including infections or kidney stones.

Blood pressure monitoring is another crucial aspect of renal health check-ups. The kidneys play a key role in regulating blood pressure by adjusting the volume of blood and the amount of sodium excreted. Hypertension can damage the blood vessels in the kidneys and impair their function over time. Regular monitoring allows for the early detection of high blood pressure, enabling interventions such as lifestyle changes or medication to prevent further kidney damage.

Imaging studies, such as ultrasounds or CT scans, may be recommended in some cases to provide a visual assessment of the kidneys. These imaging techniques can reveal abnormalities such as kidney stones, cysts, or tumors. Early detection of these issues is essential for prompt and effective management.

A renal health check-up also involves an assessment of lifestyle factors that can impact kidney health. Dietary habits, hydration levels, and exercise patterns are crucial considerations. For example, a diet high in sodium can contribute to hypertension and negatively affect renal function. Adequate hydration is essential for maintaining proper kidney function as it supports the flushing out of waste products. Lifestyle modifications based on these assessments can contribute significantly to overall renal health.

For individuals with specific risk factors, such as a family history of kidney disease or certain medical conditions like diabetes or hypertension, more frequent and targeted renal health check-ups may be recommended. Early detection and management of these risk factors can prevent or slow down the progression of kidney disease.

In conclusion, regular health check-ups focused on renal function are essential for maintaining overall well-being. These check-ups involve a combination of blood tests, urine analysis, blood pressure monitoring, imaging studies, and lifestyle assessments. Early detection of kidney issues allows for timely intervention, preventing the progression of renal diseases and ensuring optimal kidney function. Making renal health a priority through routine check-ups is a proactive step towards a healthier and more vibrant life.

Adjusting the Renal Reset Plan as Needed

The renal system plays a crucial role in maintaining the body's internal environment by regulating fluid and electrolyte balance. When the kidneys face challenges or disruptions, it becomes necessary to implement a renal reset plan to restore their optimal function. However, this plan is not a one-size-fits-all solution. It requires careful monitoring and adjustments based on individual responses and changing conditions.

The renal reset plan involves various components, including dietary modifications, fluid management, and lifestyle changes. These elements aim to support renal health, manage electrolyte imbalances, and alleviate stress on the kidneys. Despite its effectiveness, flexibility in the plan is essential to accommodate the dynamic nature of health conditions, lifestyle factors, and individual variations.

Dietary adjustments are a cornerstone of the renal reset plan. A low-sodium diet is often recommended to manage fluid balance and blood pressure. However, the extent of sodium restriction may need fine-tuning based on individual responses. Some individuals may be more sensitive to sodium intake than others, and factors such as age, overall health, and the presence of other medical conditions can influence dietary requirements.

Additionally, protein intake is a critical consideration. While reducing protein may be beneficial in certain renal conditions, it's crucial to strike a balance. In some cases, too little protein can lead to malnutrition, emphasizing the importance of personalized adjustments. Regular monitoring of renal function markers, such as blood urea nitrogen (BUN) and creatinine levels, helps gauge the impact of dietary changes and guides further adjustments.

Fluid management is another aspect that requires ongoing evaluation. Adequate hydration is essential for kidney function, but excessive fluid intake can strain the kidneys. Monitoring urine output, color, and specific gravity can provide valuable insights into hydration status. Adjustments to fluid intake should be made based on individual needs, taking into account factors like climate, physical activity, and overall health.

Pharmacological interventions are often part of the renal reset plan, and their effectiveness can vary among individuals. Regular assessment of medication responses and potential side effects is crucial. Dosages may need to be adjusted based on renal function changes, ensuring optimal therapeutic outcomes while minimizing adverse effects. Collaboration with healthcare providers is vital to fine-tune medication regimens and address any emerging concerns.

Lifestyle modifications, including exercise and stress management, contribute significantly to renal health. Regular physical activity promotes cardiovascular health, which, in turn, benefits the kidneys. However, the intensity and type of exercise should be tailored to individual capabilities and preferences. Stress reduction techniques, such as mindfulness and relaxation exercises, play a role in supporting overall well-being and may indirectly impact renal function.

Periodic medical check-ups are essential for evaluating the effectiveness of the renal reset plan. Regular monitoring of blood pressure, renal function markers, and other relevant parameters allows healthcare providers to identify emerging issues and make timely adjustments to the plan. Patient feedback and self-monitoring also play a crucial role in refining the approach, as individuals may notice subtle changes or specific triggers that need attention.

Patient education is a key component of successful renal reset plan management. Empowering individuals with knowledge about their condition, dietary guidelines, and lifestyle recommendations enhances their ability to actively participate in their healthcare. This understanding fosters a sense of ownership and encourages individuals to communicate effectively with their healthcare team, facilitating collaborative decision-making and timely adjustments to the renal reset plan.

In conclusion, adjusting the renal reset plan as needed is a dynamic and personalized process. Recognizing the individuality of responses to dietary, fluid, pharmacological, and lifestyle interventions is essential for optimizing renal health. Regular monitoring, collaboration with healthcare providers, and patient education form the foundation of a successful and adaptable renal reset plan. By embracing flexibility and tailoring interventions based on evolving needs, individuals can navigate the complexities of renal health with greater precision and efficacy.

CHAPTER 13

Celebrating Progress in renal reset

The journey of medical advancement is often marked by breakthroughs that revolutionize our understanding and treatment of various health conditions. Among these milestones, the progress in renal reset stands out as a beacon of hope for millions battling kidney-related ailments. This transformative approach to renal health has not only changed the landscape of nephrology but has also offered renewed optimism to patients and healthcare professionals alike.

Renal reset refers to a series of innovative interventions designed to restore and enhance the function of the kidneys.The kidneys are responsible for filtering waste and surplus fluids from the blood, balancing electrolytes, and regulating blood pressure.When these vital organs face dysfunction or disease, it can have severe consequences for overall health. The traditional methods of managing renal disorders often involve medication and lifestyle modifications, but renal reset takes a more proactive and sophisticated approach.

One of the groundbreaking aspects of renal reset is its focus on regenerative medicine. This field harnesses the body's own healing mechanisms to repair damaged tissues and organs. Researchers and clinicians are exploring various techniques, including stem cell therapy and tissue engineering, to stimulate kidney regeneration. By tapping into the regenerative potential of the body, renal reset holds the promise of not just managing symptoms but promoting actual healing and restoration of renal function.

In recent years, stem cell therapy has emerged as a particularly promising avenue within renal reset. Stem cells possess the unique ability to differentiate into different cell types, including those found in the kidneys. This capability opens up avenues for repairing damaged renal tissue and restoring optimal function. Clinical trials and research studies have shown encouraging results, with some patients experiencing significant improvements in kidney function after receiving stem cell treatments.

Beyond regenerative medicine, renal reset also encompasses advancements in precision medicine and personalized treatment approaches. With a deeper understanding of the genetic and molecular factors influencing kidney health, healthcare professionals can tailor interventions to individual patients. This targeted approach not only enhances treatment efficacy but also minimizes potential side effects, leading to more favorable outcomes and improved quality of life for those with renal conditions.

Furthermore, technology has played a pivotal role in advancing renal reset. Innovations such as wearable devices and remote monitoring systems enable continuous tracking of key indicators related to kidney function. This real-time data empowers both patients and healthcare providers to make informed decisions, allowing for proactive management of renal health and early detection of potential issues.

As we celebrate progress in renal reset, it's essential to acknowledge the collaborative efforts of researchers, clinicians, and the patients themselves. The journey from concept to clinical application is often long and challenging, requiring dedication, resources, and a collective commitment to advancing medical science. The stories of individuals who have benefited from renal reset highlight the transformative impact of these innovations on the lives of those grappling with renal disorders.

In conclusion, the strides made in renal reset represent a triumph of science and a beacon of hope for individuals facing kidney-related challenges. From regenerative medicine to precision treatments and technological advancements, the multifaceted approach of renal reset holds great promise for the future of nephrology. As we look ahead, the ongoing commitment to research and collaboration ensures that the journey of progress in renal reset continues, offering new possibilities and improved outcomes for renal health.

Sustaining Kidney-Friendly Habits

Maintaining kidney health is crucial for overall well-being. Adopting kidney-friendly habits can significantly contribute to the prevention of kidney-related issues. These habits encompass various aspects of lifestyle, including diet, hydration, exercise, and overall health management.

Dietary Choices:
A cornerstone of kidney-friendly habits is a balanced and mindful diet. Individuals should focus on consuming foods that promote kidney health while avoiding those that may strain the kidneys. Incorporating fruits and vegetables rich in antioxidants, such as berries, bell peppers, and leafy greens, can provide essential nutrients without overburdening the kidneys. Additionally, limiting sodium intake is vital to manage blood pressure and reduce the risk of kidney damage.

Hydration:
Adequate hydration is crucial for kidney function. Water helps flush toxins from the body and prevents the formation of kidney stones. Individuals should strive to maintain a regular and healthy fluid intake, adjusting it based on factors like climate, physical activity,

and overall health. While water is the primary choice, herbal teas and infused water can add variety to hydration routines.

Limiting Phosphorus and Potassium:
For those with kidney concerns, managing phosphorus and potassium intake is paramount. High levels of these minerals can lead to complications, particularly for individuals with kidney disease. Foods with controlled phosphorus and potassium content, such as cauliflower, cabbage, and apples, can be included in the diet to maintain a healthy balance.

Regular Exercise:
Physical activity plays a vital role in supporting overall health, including kidney function. Engaging in regular exercise promotes cardiovascular health, which, in turn, contributes to optimal kidney function. Activities like walking, swimming, or cycling can be tailored to individual fitness levels and preferences, fostering a sustainable habit that benefits the kidneys in the long run.

Monitoring Blood Pressure:
Hypertension is a leading cause of kidney damage. Regular monitoring of blood pressure and taking steps to keep it within a healthy range are essential for kidney health. This may involve medication, lifestyle modifications, and

stress management techniques. Maintaining a healthy weight, adopting a low-sodium diet, and limiting alcohol intake can contribute to blood pressure management.

Avoiding Over-the-Counter Medications:
Certain over-the-counter medications, including nonsteroidal anti-inflammatory drugs (NSAIDs), can have adverse effects on kidney function. Individuals should consult healthcare professionals before using such medications, especially if they have pre-existing kidney conditions.

Regular Health Check-ups:
Preventive healthcare measures, such as regular check-ups and screenings, play a crucial role in identifying potential kidney issues early on. Routine blood and urine tests can provide valuable insights into kidney function, allowing for timely interventions if needed.

Managing Diabetes:
For individuals with diabetes, managing blood sugar levels is paramount in preventing kidney complications. Consistent monitoring of glucose levels, medication adherence, and lifestyle modifications, including a diabetic-friendly diet, contribute to overall kidney health.

Stress Management:
Chronic stress has been shown to have a deleterious influence on general health, including renal function. Adopting stress-management techniques such as meditation, yoga, or deep-breathing exercises can help alleviate stress and contribute to kidney-friendly habits.

In conclusion, sustaining kidney-friendly habits involves a holistic approach to health and well-being. From mindful dietary choices and proper hydration to regular exercise and stress management, these habits contribute to the prevention of kidney-related issues. Incorporating these practices into daily life not only supports kidney health but also fosters overall physical and mental well-being. Always consult with healthcare professionals for personalized advice based on individual health needs and conditions.

CONCLUSION

 The "Nourishing Dietary Guide for Renal Reset" offers a transformative journey toward holistic kidney health. As readers navigate the pages of this comprehensive guide, they embark on a nuanced exploration of nutrition, understanding that nourishment extends far beyond mere sustenance. The author's meticulous research and empathetic approach illuminate the intricate relationship between dietary choices and renal well-being.

The book serves as a beacon of empowerment, empowering readers to reclaim control over their health through informed dietary decisions. It dispels myths and misconceptions, replacing them with a nuanced understanding of how various nutrients impact renal function. With each turn of the page, the reader is equipped not only with practical recipes but also with the knowledge to make personalized and sustainable dietary choices.

The narrative unfolds like a roadmap, guiding individuals through the intricacies of crafting a renal-friendly lifestyle. From insightful discussions on the role of hydration to exploring the dynamic interplay of protein, sodium, and potassium, the guide becomes a trusted companion in the reader's quest for renal well-being. It not only addresses the immediate concerns but also fosters a long-term perspective on health maintenance.

What sets this guide apart is its ability to bridge the gap between medical knowledge and everyday practices. It seamlessly weaves scientific insights into accessible language, making the complex world of renal nutrition comprehensible to a broad audience. As readers embrace the suggested dietary modifications, they embark on a journey of self-discovery, realizing the profound impact of food choices on their overall health and vitality.

The book's holistic approach extends beyond the kitchen, encouraging readers to consider lifestyle factors that contribute to renal health. From stress management techniques to the importance of regular physical activity, the guide encompasses a spectrum of practices aimed at nurturing the body and soul. It paints a vivid picture of a balanced and harmonious life where nutrition becomes a cornerstone for resilience and vitality.

In the grand tapestry of renal health, this guide emerges as a pivotal thread, weaving together the wisdom of medical science, the artistry of culinary exploration, and the resilience of the human spirit. It not only addresses the challenges posed by renal conditions but reframes them as opportunities for positive transformation. The reader is not merely a passive recipient of information but an active participant in the journey towards renewed well-being.

As the final chapter unfolds, readers find themselves equipped with more than just recipes; they possess a newfound understanding of their bodies and a sense of agency over their health destinies. The "Nourishing Dietary Guide for Renal Reset" transcends the conventional boundaries of dietary literature, leaving an indelible mark on the reader's consciousness—a call to embrace a life where nourishment becomes a conscious and compassionate act, laying the foundation for a revitalized, renal-reset future.

REVIEW PAGE

Dear valued reader, your journey through the pages of my book is a shared odyssey that I cherish deeply. Your unique perspective breathes life into the characters and narrative, making your voice an invaluable part of this literary voyage. I invite you to take a moment to reflect on the emotions, the twists, and the revelations you experienced within these chapters. Your review is not just a testament to the work, but a beacon for others yet to embark on this adventure. Share your thoughts, let your words resonate with fellow readers, and be a part of the community that enriches this literary tapestry. Your feedback is the heartbeat of this story, and I am genuinely grateful for your contribution. Thank you for being a vital part of this literary conversation, shaping the legacy of these words for future readers to come

Dear Reader,

Thank you for exploring the Nourishing Dietary Guide for Renal Reset. Your commitment to prioritizing kidney health is commendable. Embrace this transformative journey, and may the valuable insights within the book guide you towards renewed well-being. Your dedication to a nourishing lifestyle is a powerful investment in your health. Gratitude for being on this path with us!

Warm Regards
(**Candice Foster**)